Vegetables

Learn To Enjoy More Varieties While Benefitting Your Health

Healthy Food Series

By Rod Stone

Copyright Notice

Vegetables

Learn To Enjoy More Varieties While Benefitting Your Health

Part of

Healthy Food Series

Table of Contents

PREFACE

We, the people of the World have a problem.

And it's not getting any better.

We are letting big agriculture and big food providers dictate how and what we eat. This in turn is creating an unhealthy world.

In the past we not only ate our veggies, but we ate a wider variety of vegetables. By doing this we were healthier! Big agriculture and big food providers have led to more and more processed foods and "fast food meals."

This book along with others in the *Healthy Food Series* has been written to help you eat better. This book provides you with a large variety of vegetables, their nutritional values, how to pick the best quality and a few ways to use them. This along with our book on Vegetable Recipes will help you understand and use a larger variety of vegetables for a healthier life.

I am using much information provided by "the first dietitian in America" Sarah Tyson Rorer along with current updated information.

I began writing articles on health and nutrition in the mid '90s. In 2004 I started working with people and providing information and products to assist with health and nutrition. In 2008 I started to become involved with the importance of specialized high intensity workouts. In 2011 my group became involved in Universal Energy and related fields. All of this has led to my Healthy Food Series of books, which this book is the second of our group.

I have also created a website (http://vegetables.healthyfoodseries.com/) in order to provide you with pictures and additional information to improve your use of this book.

We also have a facebook page: (https://www.facebook.com/pages/Healthy-Lifestyle-Solutions/142944525806652). Here we have recipes, tips, and much more.

INTRODUCTION

The structure of the work in this book is taken from "the first dietitian in America" Sarah Tyson Rorer. The major part of the book on health benefits, selection and storage and preparation is somewhat taken from her works and a variety of other current works.

More and more studies are showing that eating more like a vegetarian makes for a healthier lifestyle.

But most people do not understand vegetables or how to prepare them for taste and nutrition. Between this book, our book on *Vegetable Recipes* and our websites (http://vegetarianrecipes.healthyfoodseries.com/) and (http://vegetables.healthyfoodseries.com/) and our facebook page https://www.facebook.com/pages/Healthy-Lifestyle-Solutions/142944525806652) we hope to help you understand vegetables, learn how to properly prepare them and start on a nutritious road to lifelong health.

This book is part of the Healthy Food Series. The Healthy Food Series is being created to help you to a better, healthier life. Every day we search for ways to feel better; this makes our days more enjoyable for ourselves as well as those around us.

We will discuss more than just healthy food as we provide you with information so that you can have a better life.

We are looking at creating a membership service that will provide you with even more detailed information.

We hope you find benefits from all of our services.

Rod Stone

IMPORTANCE OF VEGETABLES

Did you know these facts?

- Vegetarian foods are a major source of nutrition for most people in the world.
- Vegetarians have lower rates of heart disease and some forms of cancer than non-vegetarians.

Health benefits of eating vegetables:

- Eating a diet rich in vegetables and fruits as part of an overall healthy diet may reduce risk for heart disease, including heart attack and stroke.
- Eating a diet rich in some vegetables and fruits as part of an overall healthy diet may protect against certain types of cancers.
- Diets rich in foods containing fiber, such as some vegetables and fruits, may reduce the risk of heart disease, obesity, and type 2 diabetes.
- Eating vegetables and fruits rich in potassium as part of an overall healthy diet may lower blood pressure, and may also reduce the risk of developing kidney stones and help to decrease bone loss.
- Eating foods such as vegetables that are lower in calories per cup instead of some other higher-calorie food may be useful in helping to lower calorie intake

Nutrition benefits:

- Vegetables, like fruits, are low in fat but contain good amounts of vitamins and minerals. All the Green-Yellow-Orange vegetables are rich sources of calcium, magnesium, potassium, iron, beta-carotene, vitamin B-complex, vitamin-C, vitamin A, and vitamin K.

- As in fruits, vegetables too are home for many antioxidants that; firstly, help protect the human body from oxidant stress, diseases and cancers, and secondly; help the body develop the capacity to fight against these by boosting immunity.

- Additionally, vegetables are packed with soluble as well as insoluble dietary fiber known as non-starch polysaccharides (NSP) such as cellulose, mucilage, hemi-cellulose, gums, pectin...etc. These substances absorb excess water in the colon, retain a good amount of moisture in the fecal matter, and help its smooth passage out of the body. Thus, sufficient fiber offers protection from conditions like hemorrhoids, colon cancer, chronic constipation, and rectal fissures.

- Dietary fiber from vegetables, as part of an overall healthy diet, helps reduce blood cholesterol levels and may lower risk of heart disease. Fiber is important for proper bowel function. It helps reduce constipation and diverticulosis. Fiber-containing foods such as vegetables help provide a feeling of fullness with fewer calories.

- Vegetables have no cholesterol.

- Vegetables are important sources of many nutrients, including potassium, dietary fiber, folate (folic acid), vitamin A, and vitamin C.
- Diets rich in potassium may help to maintain healthy blood pressure. Vegetable sources of potassium include sweet potatoes, white potatoes, white beans, tomato products (paste, sauce, and juice), beet greens, soybeans, lima beans, spinach, lentils, and kidney beans.
- Folate (folic acid) helps the body form red blood cells. Women of childbearing age who may become pregnant should consume adequate folate from foods, and in addition 400 mcg of synthetic folic acid from fortified foods or supplements. This reduces the risk of neural tube defects, spina bifida, and anencephaly during fetal development.
- Vitamin A keeps eyes and skin healthy and helps to protect against infections.
- Vitamin C helps heal cuts and wounds and keeps teeth and gums healthy. Vitamin C aids in iron absorption.

The American people, as a class, in their rushing and bustling life, prefer to take their nitrogen from animal products, which are rather more easily digested and assimilated than vegetables. It is a fact, however, that all the elements necessary for the building of the body are found in the vegetable world. Our working animals, "beasts of burden," build and repair large bodies, under heavy labor, on materials from the vegetable kingdom.

True, their digestive apparatus is rather different from man's, and is better suited to the dry, concentrated cereals. We do not, however, get from the animal a single element except that which the animal has taken from the vegetable world. His flesh is the result of the digestion of vegetable materials. Flesh is living tissue, the partly digested food, hence, more easily digested by man than vegetables at first hand. Meat is rich in water, containing less nitrogen than peas, beans and lentils, but in a more acceptable form to many people.

Vegetables, as well as animal foods, contain nitrogenous substances. Fats are well represented, and while they resemble in chemical composition the animal fats, the fact remains that they produce less heat on combustion. They contain more olein and less of the solid components. To the vegetable kingdom we look for our carbohydrates, sugars and starches — both difficult materials to cook well. The remaining constituents, mineral salts, have great dietetic importance; they are easily dissolved and lost in cooking. Potash in green vegetables is more abundant than soda; rice, however, contains a liberal allowance of the latter. Use salt with green vegetables and potatoes, but not with rice. Vegetable foods are recommended to persons with gouty diathesis and those inclined to uric acid conditions or rheumatism. Vegetable proteids do not yield uric acid.

The true vegetarian uses all forms of vegetable foods; he does not try to live upon potatoes and so-called green or succulent vegetables. These do not contain nitrogen, and are insufficient to sustain life. Nuts well prepared and mixed with cereals, and such easily digested foods as rice give sustaining power not attainable by meat. Health and nutrition depend entirely upon the class of vegetables selected. We are seeing world wide the health benefits of eating more and a variety of vegetables.

Meat carefully cooked is more easily digested than some vegetables; but vegetables are clean and wholesome. Nitrogenous vegetables are slow of digestion; hence, the vegetarian requires but two meals per day; but in those two meals, especially if his diet is well selected, he will receive more nourishment than from three meals of meat. Two points have been gained, time spent in eating and money saved. Then, too, he has had much greater variety. The vegetarian is not compelled to eat steaks, chops and roasted beef to be followed by roasts of beef, steaks and chops; but selects from a score of dishes made by blending different vegetables, nuts and fruits. Vegetable foods are not to any great extent digested in the stomach, with the exception of the leguminous seeds, which are rich in proteids. Vegetable foods call forth greater mechanical effort on the part of the stomach than meats. If a person has indigestion, meats are to be preferred. The amount of cellulose or waste in vegetable foods keeps up the peristaltic motion of the intestines and lower bowels; hence, vegetable eaters are very rarely troubled with constipation and torpid livers. Skin diseases are frequently due to a lack of green vegetables.

Today, most people focus on fast foods, meats and all types of processed foods. Many people preparing meals are not properly trained in how to prepare foods in general and especially vegetables.

Badly cooked vegetables are tasteless; all the flavor has been cooked out and poured down the drain. Potatoes, a common vegetable, served in nearly every household once or twice a day, are seldom well cooked, palatable or sightly. Rice is almost unfit for food; in nine cases out of ten it is heavy and sodden, a mass of wet starch.

Vegetables are divided into four classes: Those rich in nitrogen, muscle and tissue building foods; those containing carbohydrates, starch and sugar; fatty vegetables, nuts and olives; and the vegetables containing water and mineral matter. In the first class we have peas, beans and lentils, and the chick pea of the East. Nitrogen is also found in goodly quantities in the cereals and nuts and glutin macaroni. In the second class, carbohydrates, we have rice, white bread, potatoes, the ordinary macaroni. Those containing mineral matter and water are the so-called succulent vegetables, as cabbage, carrots, turnips, spinach, cress, lettuce and tomatoes. The nitrogenous principles of vegetables are acted upon in the stomach the same as those of meat; the carbohydrates in the mouth and the small intestines; fats are emulsionized by the secretions from the pancreas and gall. There is no difference between meats and vegetables in the place or method of digestion. The effects upon the body, the time consumed, and the mechanical efforts of the body are, no doubt, radically different.

BOTANICAL CLASSIFICATION OF OUR
COMMON VEGETABLES

Dicotyledons.

Cruciferae, Mustard Family.
Water-cress; Horseradish; Cabbage tribe; Turnip; Rutabaga; Mustard, black and white; Peppergrass; Radish.

Capparidaceae, Caper Family.
Capers.

Malvaceae, Mallow Family.
Okra.

Geraniaceae, Geranium Family.
Wood Sorrel, Nasturtium.

Leguminosae, Pulse Family.
Soy Bean; Peanut; Kidney Bean; String Bean; Lima Bean; Black Bean; Pea; Chick Pea; Lentil; St. John's Bread.

Cucurbitaceae, Gourd Family.
Pumpkin; Squash, summer and winter; Cucumber; Vegetable Marrow.

Umbelliferae, Parsley Family.
This family contains many of the aromatic seeds. Carrot; Coriander; Sweet Cicely; Fennel; Celery; Celeriac; Caraway; Parsley; Angelica; Parsnip.

Valerianaceae, Valerian Family.
Corn Salad.

Compositae, Composite Family.

Jerusalem Artichoke; Globe Artichoke; Cardoon; Chicory; Endive; Salsify; Dandelion; Lettuce; Romaine.

Convolvulaceae, Convolvulus Family.
Sweet Potato.

Solanaceae, Nightshade Family.
Tomato; White Potato; Egg Plant; Chilli Pepper, in all its varieties.

Labiatae, Mint Family.
The leaves of the plants of this family arc aromatic. Sweet Basil; Mint; Savory; Marjoram; Thyme; Sage; Stachys.

Chenopodiaceae, Goosefoot Family.
Spinach; Beet.

Phytolaccaceae, Poke-weed Family.
Poke or Scoke.

Polygonaceae, Buckwheat Family.
Dock; Sorrel; Buckwheat.

Lauraceae, Laurel Family. (This is not the family to which the mountain and sheep laurel belong.)
Sassafras; Bay-leaves.

Monocotyledons.

Scitamineae, Banana Family.
Ginger; Arrowroot; Tous-les-mois; Banana.

Dioscoreaceae, Yam Family.
Yam.

Liliaceae, Lily Family.

Asparagus; Onion; Leek; Garlic; Scullion; Chives; Shallots.

Palmaceae, Palm Family.
    Sago (Dates and Cocoanuts also).

Gramineae, Grass Family.
    Rice; Oats; Wheat; Rye; Barley; Maize; Sorghum; Durra or Kaffir Corn; Millet.

Of the many thousands of flowerless plants but few are used as food. In the Orient the young fronds of the common brake are used as a green vegetable, while the rhizomes are used as a source of starch.

Some of the sea-weeds have proved valuable in periods of scarcity, while the Irish moss and dulse are used at all times.

Many lichens have been used as dyes, but very few as food. Arctic explorers have sometimes been forced to eat various plants of this group. The best known lichen, however, is the Iceland moss.

All the mushrooms and truffles belong to the large group of fungi plants void of chlorophyll.

PREPARING VEGETABLES

All green vegetables should be freshly gathered, washed well in cold water, and cooked in freshly-boiled water until tender, no longer. After water has boiled for a time it parts with its gases and becomes hard, and most vegetables are better cooked in soft water. It is a well-known fact that split peas, dried beans and lentils do not boil soft in hard water. The salts of lime, sulphate or gypsum coagulate the casein which these seeds contain. In some cases, however, the solvent power of pure, soft water is so great that it destroys the firmness, color and outside covering (skin) of the green vegetables, and allows their juices to pass out into the water. This is especially true of green peas and beans. In these cases, therefore, hard water is better than soft. A teaspoonful of common salt added to every gallon of water hardens it at once. A half-teaspoonful of bi-carbonate of soda to every gallon of water renders it soft. French books recommend the same quantity of carbonate of ammonia for the latter purpose.

Vegetables, as a rule, should be cooked in uncovered vessels, covering does not keep in the flavor. Rapid boiling renders underground vegetables, as parsnips, carrots and turnips, tough. Cook them in water at 210° Fahr.; this softens the fibre and quickly renders them tender, and at the same time, they retain their flavor and color. Rapid boiling dissipates the flavor and spoils the color.

Rice and macaroni should be boiled rapidly, not that the water is hotter, but the motion of rapidly boiling water washes apart and separates the particles. Both contain starch; if allowed to simmer or cooked in a double boiler, they become soft, sticky, water-soaked and soggy. Potatoes must be cooked at the boiling point.

Young, green vegetables should be cooked in boiling salted water. Onions, if boiled in pure, soft water, are almost tasteless, and all the after-salting cannot restore to them the sweet saline taste and the strong aroma which they possess when boiled in hard water (salted). If green vegetables are wilted, soak them for an hour or two in clear, cold water; never add salt, as it hardens the tissues.

Peas, beans and lentils are the most nutritious of all vegetable substances. They are said to contain as much carbon (heat -giving food) as wheat, and almost double the amount of nitrogen (muscle-forming food). The nitrogenous element of these vegetables consists chiefly of vegetable casein.

Lentils afford the most concentrated form of vegetable diet, and in olden times their nutritious value was fully appreciated. Esau sold his birthright for a mess of red lentil pottage. We read that the Pyramids were built by men who lived on lentils, garlic and water. A dish served to persons of distinction in the time of Pharaoh was composed of lentils, and with this high reputation they are almost unknown in this country, except to the Germans, who use them for soup, which, though made entirely without meat, is most nutritious.

It is said that all vegetables not containing starch are best and more wholesome served raw. The roots, as turnips, carrots and beets, must, however, be grated or scraped. The dense fibre renders them difficult of mastication and digestion.

A GROUP OF STARCHY VEGETABLES

Photos can be found at:
http://vegetables.healthyfoodseries.com/starchy-vegetables/

Potatoes
Rice
Yams
Hominy
Tapioca
Hominy grits
Sago
Italian pastes in general, as vermicelli, macaroni, spaghetti
Cassava
Arrowroot
Chestnuts
Tous-les-mois
Lotus

This group contains all vegetables common to the United States, in which starch is the principal nutrient, and the cereals, chestnuts, and manufactured foods, as macaroni, etc., served as vegetables.

Starchy vegetables belonging to the carbohydrates are fat formers, and heat and energy producers.

They are digested in the mouth and small intestines; unless well masticated in the small intestine only.

POTATOES

(Solanum tuberosum, Linnaeus)

The portion of the plant used as food constitutes the tuber, an enlarged, or gorged, underground stem — the store-house for nourishment for the young plants.

Many varieties, quite dissimilar in composition and general appearance, are grown in different parts of the world. Those grown in South America are of a rich yellow color when cooked, and much more dry and mealy than those grown in the United States. The German potatoes, imported for salads, are small, slightly yellow, dry and sweet. These are sold at ten cents per quart at the German delicatessen in all large cities. They are much better for salad than the American varieties.

Potatoes should be kept for winter use in a cool, dry, dark place. Warmth, light and moisture cause growth and loss of nutrition, while they increase the quantity of solanin, a poisonous substance found in all potatoes. This substance is in greater quantity in very young and old potatoes. Those ripe, or full grown, contain least, but in all cases it is dissipated or driven off in the cooking. Water in which potatoes have been boiled is unsafe for food; it should be thrown away. In making potato soup, par-boil the potatoes for five minutes and throw away the water. The water of the second boiling is usually free from solanin and quite safe. Pare sparingly, as both nourishment and mineral matter are greater near the skin. Observe a cross section of a good full-grown potato; first comes the skin, then the fibro-vascular bundles, a narrow white layer, rich in starch and mineral matter, then the fleshy portion, in the centre of which is a watery core. The fibro-vascular layer contains nearly as much nourishment as the remaining portion of the potato.

As the nutritious part lies near the skin, peel as thin as possible and throw each potato into cold water as soon as pared. Select potatoes of the same size for cooking, all the large potatoes should be cooked at one time, medium sized at another, and the small ones at another. As the starch cells are thicker around the outside, the cutting of a large potato to make it correspond in size to the smaller ones, allows the water to penetrate and the potato becomes sodden and heavy. Potatoes boiled in their jackets are without doubt better than those that are pared. The saline constituents of the potato are potash, and when potatoes are pared a large percentage of these salts, which are freely soluble in water, are drawn out into the water, and the potato has rather a flat taste. This also contradicts the idea of a ' simple paring around the potato. The salts dissolve out if the skin is broken.

Carefully cooked they constitute a wholesome and easily digested starchy food. The amount of nitrogen is small, and does not belong to the flesh forming proteids. Potatoes cannot be depended upon as a complete food, but should be served with such nitrogenous foods as nuts, peas, beans, lentils, or lean meats. The food value and digestibility, however, depend entirely on the method of cooking. Baked, or boiled, mealy, not heavy, they are rather more easily digested than white bread or hominy; when fried or mashed and patted down with butter, served in a covered dish, they are less digestible. When fried, covered with grease, the primary digestion, which is in the mouth, is lost, as each grain of starch is surrounded by fat. The saliva cannot penetrate the fat in the usual time given to mastication, which leaves the entire digestion to the intestines; the stomach has little or no action on potatoes.

Composition of Potatoes

```
Water . . . . . . . . . . . . . . . . . . . . . 75.0
Albuminoids . . . . . . . . . . . . . . . . 1.2
Extractives, as solanin and organic acids 1.5
Starch . . . . . . . . . . . . . . . . . . . 18.0
Dextrin and pectose . . . . . . . . . . .  2.0
Fat  . . . . . . . . . . . . . . . . . . . .  0.3
Cellulose . . . . . . . . . . . . . . . . .  1.0
Mineral matter . . . . . . . . . . . . . .  1.0
```

Very new and very old potatoes are scarcely worth the cooking. A potato sprouts at the expense of the starch, nearest the skin, hence, the potato withers, and the nutrition is lost. Old potatoes should be pared and soaked in cold water at least thirty minutes before cooking. Full grown potatoes do not require soaking.

Potatoes belong to the carbohydrates, fat and energy producers, and are digested principally in the small intestine.

Health Benefits:

- Potatoes are one of the richest sources of starch, vitamins, minerals and dietary fiber. They contain very little fat and no cholesterol.

- They are very good natural sources of both soluble and insoluble fiber. The dietary fiber in them increases the bulk of the stool, thus, it helps prevent constipation, decrease absorption of dietary cholesterol and there by lower plasma LDL cholesterol. Additionally, the rich fiber content also helps protect from colon polyps and cancer.

- The fiber content aids in slow digestion starch and absorption of simple sugars in the gut. It thus help keep blood sugar levels within the normal range and avoid wide fluctuations. For the same reason, potato is considered as reliable source of carbohydrates in diabetics.

- The tubers are one of the richest sources of B-complex group of vitamins such as pyridoxine (vitamin B6), thiamin, niacin, pantothenic acid and folates.

- Fresh potato along with its skin is good source of antioxidant vitamin; vitamin-C. Regular consumption of foods rich in vitamin-C helps body develop resistance against infectious agents and scavenge harmful, pro-inflammatory free radicals.

- They also contain adequate amounts of many essential minerals like Iron, manganese, magnesium, phosphorous, copper and potassium.

- Red and *russet potatoes* contain good amount vitamin A, and antioxidant flavonoids like carotenes and zeaxanthins.
- Recent studies at Agricultural research service (by plant genetics scientist Roy Navarre) suggests that flavonoid antioxidant, *quercetin* present in potatoes has anti-cancer and cardio-protective properties.

Selection and storage:

Fresh potatoes are readily available in the stores everywhere. Look for tubers that feature firm in texture and have smooth waxy, instead of dry, surface. They normally have numerous "eyes" on their surface. Avoid those that feature soft in hand, have slumpy appearance, with cuts, patches and bruises.

Oftentimes, you may come across greenish discoloration with sprouts over their surface. Do not buy them since the discoloration is indication of outdated stock and formation of toxic alkaloid *solanine.*

At home, they should be stored in cool, dry and dark place. Exposure to sunlight and excess moisture will cause potatoes to sprout and to form toxic alkaloid solanine.

Preparation:

Being a root vegetable they often subjected to infestation and therefore wash them thoroughly before cooking. Fresh, cleaned tubers can be enjoyed with skin to derive benefits of fiber and vitamins.

Skin-on or peeled, whole or cut up, with seasonings or without. The potato can be used in many ways.

Mashed potatoes – first boiled and peeled, and then masked with milk or yogurt and butter.

Whole baked, boiled or steamed.

French-fried potatoes or chips.

Prepare delicious soup or chowder with leeds, corn, onion and seasonings.

Cut into cubes and roasted; scalloped, diced or sliced and fried.

Grated and prepare dumplings, and pancakes.

Safety Precaution:

Potatoes may contain toxic alkaloids, *solanine* and *chaconine*. These alkaloids present in the greatest concentrations just underneath the skin and increase proportionately with age and exposure to sun light. Cooking at high temperatures (over 170 °C) partly destroys these toxic substances.

When consumed in sufficient amounts, these compounds may cause headache, weakness, muscle cramps and, in severe cases loss of consciousness and coma; however, poisoning from potatoes occurs very rarely. Exposure to light also causes green discoloration; thus giving a visual clue as areas of the tuber that may have more toxins; however, this does not provide a definitive clue, as greening and solanine accumulation can occur independently to each other. Some varieties contain greater solanine concentrations than others.

RICE

(*Oryza sativa*, Linn.)

Rice belongs to the great grass order, the group of cereals. It is exceedingly rich in starch, and contains a small amount of proteid, fat, and mineral matter. It is said, however, that varieties of the East Indian rice contain more nitrogenous constituents than the rice grown in America. In boiling, rice parts with a goodly quantity of both starch and mineral matter, hence, the necessity of steaming it in small quantities of water, East Indian fashion, or saving the water in which it is boiled for soups.

Rice is highly valuable as a starchy food, containing four times as much nourishment as potatoes, and requires only one hour for perfect digestion. It is readily absorbed and leaves little or no waste in the intestines. From both a money and nutritive standpoint it is the most desirable starchy food to serve with nitrogenous materials, as meats, eggs and milk. It forms the staple food for three-fourths of the world's inhabitants.

An ancient grain that has been cultivated for centuries. Rice is commercially classified by size: long, medium or short grain. Long-grain rice is 4-5 times its width and is available in white and brown varieties, which are light, dry grains that separate easily when cooked. Basmati rice is a perfumy East Indian variety of long-grain rice.

Short-grain rice has fat, almost round grains that have a higher starch content. When cooked, it tends to be quite moist and viscous, causing the grains to stick together. Also called pearl rice or glutinous rice (although it's gluten-free). Other varieties of short-grain rice are Arborio and Mochi.

Medium-grain rice has a size and character in between the other two.

Rice can be further divided into two other broad categoriess: brown and white. Brown rice is the entire grain with only the inedible outer husk removed. The nutritious, high-fiber bran coating gives it a light tan color, nutlike flavor and chewy texture. Brown rice takes slightly longer to cook. White rice has had the husk, bran and germ removed. Regular white rice is sometimes referred to as polished rice. For converted or parboiled white rice, the unhulled grain has been soaked, pressure-steamed and dried. Converted rice has a pale beige cast and takes slightly longer to cook than regular white rice. Instant or quick white rice has been fully or partially cooked before being dehydrated and packaged.

COMPOSITION OF DRY RICE

Water 14.6
Albuminoids, etc 7.5

Starch, etc. 76.0
Fat 0.5
Cellulose 0.9
Mineral matter 0.5

COMPOSITION OF BOILED RICE

Water 52.7
Proteid 5.0
Fat 0.1
Carbo-hydrates 41.9
Mineral matter 0.3

Rice is a carbohydrate, a fat forming and an energy producing food, and digested principally in the small intestine.

Health Benefits:

The health benefits of rice include its ability to provide fast and instant energy, regulate and improve bowel movements, stabilize blood sugar levels, and slow down the aging process, while also providing an essential source of vitamin B1 to the human body. Other benefits include its ability to boost skin health, increase the metabolism, aid in digestion, reduce high blood pressure, help weight loss efforts, improve the immune system and provide protection against dysentery, cancer, and heart disease. Rice is a fundamental food in many cultural cuisines around the world, and it is an important cereal crop that feeds more than half of the world's population.

The various benefits of rice can be found in more than forty thousand varieties of this cereal that is available throughout the world. The two main categories are whole grain rice and white rice. Whole grain rice is not processed very much, so it is high in nutritional value, whereas white rice is processed so that the bran or outer covering is removed, leaving it with less nutritional value. People choose different styles of rice for particular flavors, depending on their culinary needs, the availability, and the potential for healthy benefits as well!

Great Source of Energy: Since rice is abundant in carbohydrates, it acts as fuel for the body and aids in the normal functioning of the brain. Carbohydrates are essential to be metabolized by the body and turned into functional, usable energy. The vitamins, minerals, and various organic components increase the functioning and metabolic activity of all your organ systems, which further increases energy levels.

Cholesterol Free: Eating rice is extremely beneficial for your health, simply because it does not contain harmful fats, cholesterol or sodium. It forms an integral part of balanced diet. Any food that can provide nutrients without having any negative impacts on health is a bonus! Low levels of fat, cholesterol, and sodium will also help reduce obesity and the health conditions associated with being overweight. Rice is one of the most widely used and eaten foods in the world because it can keep people healthy and alive, even in very small quantities.

Blood Pressure Management: Rice is low in sodium, so it is considered one of the best foods for those suffering from high blood pressure and hypertension. Sodium can cause veins and arteries to constrict, increasing the stress and strain on the cardiovascular system as the blood pressure increases. This is also associated with heart conditions like atherosclerosis, heart attacks, and strokes, so avoiding excess sodium is always a good idea.

Cancer Prevention: Whole grain rice like brown rice is rich in insoluble fiber that can protect against many types of cancer. Many scientists and researchers believe that such insoluble fibers are vital for protecting the body against the development and metastasis of cancerous cells. Fiber, specifically is beneficial in defending against colorectal and intestinal cancer. However, besides fiber, rice also has natural antioxidants like vitamin C, vitamin-A, phenolic and flavonoid compounds, which also act as or stimulate antioxidants to scour the body for free radicals. Free radicals are byproducts of cellular metabolism that can do serious damage to your organ systems and cause the mutation of healthy cells into cancerous ones. Boosting your antioxidant levels is a great idea, and eating more rice is a wonderful way to do that.

Skin care: Medical experts say that powdered rice can be applied topically to cure certain skin ailments. On the Indian subcontinent, rice water is readily prescribed by ayurvedic practitioners as an effective ointment to cool off inflamed skin surfaces. The phenolic compounds that are found in rice, particularly in brown or wild rice, have anti-inflammatory properties, so they are also good for soothing irritation and redness. Whether consumed or topically applied, substance derived from rice tend to relieve a number of skin conditions. The antioxidant capacity also helps delay the appearance of wrinkles and other premature signs of aging that can affect the skin.

Alzheimer's Disease: Brown rice is said to contain high levels of nutrients that stimulate the growth and activity of neurotransmitters, subsequently helping to prevent Alzheimer's disease to a considerable extent. Various species of wild rice have been shown to stimulate neuroprotective enzymes in the brain, which inhibit the effects of free radicals and other dangerous toxins that can cause dementia and Alzheimer's disease.

Diuretic and Digestive Qualities: The husk part of rice is considered to be an effective medicine to treat dysentery, and some people say that a three month old rice plant's husks are said to have diuretic properties. Chinese people believe that rice considerably increases appetite, cures stomach ailments and reduces all digestive problems. As a diuretic, rice husk can help you lose excess water weight, eliminate toxins from the body like uric acid, and even lose weight, since approximately 4% of urine is actually made up of body fat! The high fiber content also increases bowel movement regularity and protects against various types of cancer, as well as reducing the chances of cardiovascular diseases.

Rich in Vitamins: Rice is an excellent source of vitamins and minerals like niacin, vitamin D, calcium, fiber, iron, thiamine and riboflavin. These vitamins provide the foundation for body metabolism, immune system health, and general functioning of the organ systems, since vitamins are commonly consumed in the most essential activities in the body.

Cardiovascular Health: Rice bran oil is known to have antioxidant properties that promote cardiovascular strength by reducing cholesterol levels in the body. We have already spoken about the cardiovascular benefits of fiber, and low levels of fat and sodium. Wild rice and brown rice varieties are far better than white rice in this category, since the husk of the grain is where much of the nutrients are; the husk is removed in white rice preparation.

Resistant starch: Rice abounds in resistant starch, which reaches the bowels in an undigested form. This type of starch stimulates the growth of useful bacteria that help with normal bowel movements. Also, this insoluble rice is very useful in reducing the effects of conditions like Irritable Bowel Syndrome (IBS), and diarrhea.

HOMINY
CORN (ZeaMays)

Of this we have two sorts, one almost the entire grain with the hull taken off, the other the grain ground after the hull has been removed; the latter is known as hominy grits. This is frequently served as a breakfast food, but may be served as a vegetable in place of potatoes or rice at dinner or supper. It is more easily digested boiled in water than milk. Both kinds of hominy should be soaked in cold water over night, then cooked slowly for a long while. According to

Payne the following is the correct analysis of these dried materials:

Nitrogenous matter 12.50
Starch 67.55
Dextrin 4.00
Fatty matter 8.80
Cellulose 5.90
Mineral matter 1.25

TARO

(*Colocasia antiquorum, Schott,* Variety *esculenta*)
Root of the Elephant Ear

The Sandwich Islanders make the famous poi by boiling and baking the taro root, beating it until light and allowing it to ferment for two or three days.

CASSAVA AND TAPIOCA

Both of these are very rich in starch, containing from 83 to 85%. They are made from the fleshy roots of two species of the tropical genus Manihot, one being the sweet and the other bitter. The latter, however, is used only in cases of necessity and is then robbed of its poisonous qualities by washing and drying. In manufacture, the root of the sweet variety is washed and scraped, grated and beaten to a pulp. The mass is then subjected to pressure to express the juice, which, when evaporated, gives cassava starch and tapioca. The compressed residue is cassava meal, from which cassava bread is made. Ground tapioca is sold under the name of granulated or instantaneous tapioca. "Rolled tapioca" is simply rolled before the mass of starch is quite dry. The object in grinding or rolling is to give shorter time for cooking. The large tapioca requires both long soaking and careful cooking to be at all palatable or digestible. Pearl tapioca is ground, then moistened and rolled into the shape in which it is sold.

Cassava:

Health Benefits:
- Cassava has nearly twice the calories of potatoes, perhaps highest for any tropical starch rich tubers and roots. 100 g root provides 160 calories.
- Cassava is very low in fats and protein. Nonetheless, it has more protein than that of other tropical food sources like yam, potato, plantains, etc.
- As in other roots and tubers, cassava is free from gluten. Gluten-free starch is used in special food preparations for celiac disease patients.
- Young tender cassava (yuca) leaves are a good source of dietary proteins and vitamin K. Vitamin-K has a potential role in bone mass building by promoting osteotrophic activity in the bones. It also has established role in the treatment of

Alzheimer's disease patients by limiting neuronal damage in the brain.

- Cassava is a moderate source of some of the valuable B-complex group of vitamins such as folates, thiamin, pyridoxine (vitamin B-6), riboflavin, and pantothenic acid.
- The root is the chief source of some important minerals like zinc, magnesium, copper, iron, and manganese for many inhabitants in the tropical belts. In addition, it has adequate amounts of potassium. Potassium is an important component of cell and body fluids that help regulate heart rate and blood pressure.

Selection and storage:

Cassava roots are readily available in the markets year round. Buy well-formed, hard, cylindrical root that is heavy for its size. Cleaned, and processed yuca available in the US markets, usually imported from the Central America is generally waxed, and therefore, appears bright and shiny.

Avoid old stocks, as they are out of flavor and less appetizing. Do not buy if the tubers feature cuts, breaks in the skin. Also, avoid those with mold, soft spots, and blemishes.

Fresh roots can be kept at room temperature for about 5-7 days. However, peeled and cut sections should be placed in cold water and stored in the refrigerator for up to three days.

Preparation:

In order to make yuca safe to eat, boil the cut sections in water with sea salt added for about 10-15 minutes, until tender. Drain the water before using them in various cooking recipes.

Cassava tubers are popular ingredients in fries, stew-fries, soups, and savory dishes.

Cassava sections are fried in oil until brown and crisp and served with oil, salt and pepper.

The cassava is sieved to prepare white pearls (tapioca-starch). The pearls are used in sweet pudding, savory fritters, etc.

Cassava flout is used along with yams to make fufu (polenta), which is then savored with stews.

Cassava chips and flakes are eaten as a snack.

SAGO

True sago is a pure starch made from the central part of several varieties of palms. This portion of the tree is ground, washed and strained through fine sieves. The starch is allowed to settle and again washed, dried and ground. In some parts of the East Indies, a starchy meal is made from the Cycas which must not be confounded with true sago. Pearl sago is made by mixing water with the dry starch and granulating by motion, while the mixture is drying.

Recipes for the cooking of sago will be found under desserts.

ARROWROOT

Genuine arrowroot is made from the root stalks of the *Maranta Arundinacea*, Linn. Arrowroot is the smallest of all starch granules; under the microscope it resembles closely, with the exception of the size, the potato starch. Brazilian arrowroot is frequently adulterated with potato or other inferior starches. Adulterations can be easily detected, however, by microscopic observations. Arrowroot is most easily digested of all starches and cooks at the lowest temperature. In thin gruel, the starch grains rupture at 180° Fahr.

TOUS-LES-MOIS

This is made from the tuber of *Canna edulis*, and, like arrowroot, is very easy of digestion, and cooks at about the same temperature. These are the largest of all starch grains, are round, with concentric markings and a central hilum. This starch is not used to any extent in the United States except by the Turks, who make from it a sort of jelly-like, elastic candy, called Turkish Delight.

COMMON MILLET

Millet is the seed of a plant belonging to the grass family and stands midway between wheat and rice. It is not used in the United States as human food, except by a few Germans and Russians, as a thickening of clear soups.

The Sorgho grass or East India millet, called dhoora, is very similar.

COMPOSITION

Water 13.0
Albuminoids, etc. 12.9
Fat 3.6
Carbo-hydrates 65.4
Cellulose 3.5
Mineral matter 1.6

ITALIAN PASTES

MACARONI

Italian macaroni has about the same food value as common white bread; it contains both carbonaceous and nitrogenous principles; leaning towards the first is fat, heat and force food. The primary digestion begins in the mouth, the nitrogenous principles are digested in the stomach, the starchy portion finished in the intestines. At dinner the Italian pastes take the place of potatoes or rice; when cooked with cheese and tomatoes, or milk and egg, they make admirable luncheon or supper dishes.

Macaroni with cheese forms an almost typical food. It is the bread and meat of the Italian laborer; even at hard work he finds it a satisfying and perfect diet. A few years ago the best grades were imported, but now many of the domestic articles are superior to those coming from across the water. Until within the past few years, macaroni was prepared only as a luxury for the tables of the very rich. Even now it is sparingly used throughout the country by the American laboring classes. There is no reason, however, considering its price and the ease with which it is prepared, why it should not enter extensively into the food of all our people. It is nutritious, palatable, sightly and much more easily prepared than many of our every-day dishes. It frequently lacks flavor, due, of course, to the careless manner of cooking; and this may be one reason why it is so little used. The thoughtless cook throws it into water that is not hot; simmers it gently until it is soft and pasty; drains it, pours over it a little cream sauce, puts a thick layer of chopped cheese on top, and bakes it in the oven. It comes to the table a mass of heavy paste. The cheese is hard and scorched, and all in all, it is a very uninteresting dish. Sir Henry Thompson tells us that "glutin macaroni, weight for weight, may be regarded not less valuable in the economy than beef or mutton." Served with cheese it is an admirable substitute for meat.

Glutin macaroni has meat value, and may be cooked after these same rules, allowing thirty minutes for the first cooking and at least twenty for the second.

Serve macaroni with roasted duck, birds or braised beef.

Serve spaghetti alone as a vegetable course, or with braised or roasted beef.

LOTUS

Crunchy, delicate flavored lotus root is an under-water edible rhizome of lotus plant. Since centuries, the lotus rhizome has held high esteem in oriental regions, especially in Chinese and Japanese cultures. Almost all the parts of the plant: root, young flower stalks, and seeds are being used in the cuisine.

Lotus root is grown as annual root vegetable crop in customized ponds. Although lotus can be raised from the seeds, commercially, the rhizomes with meristems (growing points) are preferred for cultivation since it takes less time for crop production. Rhizome activity in the plant usually coincides with the appearance of large floating leaves about 5-6 months after implantation.

The rhizomes grow underwater in mud. They are actually modified tubers storing energy in the form of starch. The rhizome develops into sausage-like three to five jointed nodes of about 2-4 feet length. Each rhizome segment features smooth, grey-white color and measure about 10-20 cm in length, 6-10 cm in diameter. Internally, the root has white, crunchy flesh with mild sweet, water chestnut like flavor. The cut sections reveal visually appealing display of symmetrically arranged air canals (holes) traversing along the length of the root.

The lotus fruit is an enlarged receptacle akin to sunflower head where in numerous edible seeds embedded in its head.

Health Benefits:
- Lotus root is one of the moderate calorie root vegetables. Nevertheless, it composed of several health benefiting phyto-nutrients, minerals, and vitamins.
- Lotus rhizome is very good source dietary fibers. The fiber, together with slow digesting complex carbohydrates in the root help reduce blood cholesterol, sugar, body weight and constipation conditions.
- Lotus root is one of the excellent sources of vitamin C. Vitamin C is a powerful water soluble anti-oxidant. It is required for the collagen synthesis in the body. Collagen is the main structural protein in the body required for maintaining the integrity of blood vessels, skin, organs, and bones. Regular consumption of foods rich in vitamin C helps the body protect from scurvy, develop resistance against viral infection, boosts immunity, hasten wound healing and remove cancer causing harmful free radicals from the body.
- In addition, it contains moderate levels of some of valuable B-complex group of vitamins such as pyridoxine (vitamin B-6), folates, niacin, riboflavin, pantothenic acid, and thiamin.

Pyridoxine (vitamin B-6) acts as a coenzyme in the neuro-chemical synthesis in the brain which influences mood. Adequate pyridoxine levels help control nervous irritability, headache, and tension. It also protects heart-attack risk by controlling harmful homocysteine levels in the blood.

- Further, the root provides healthy amounts of some important minerals like copper, iron, zinc, magnesium, and manganese. Copper is a cofactor for many vital enzymes, including *cytochrome c-oxidase* and *superoxide dismutase* (other minerals function as cofactors for this enzyme are manganese and zinc). Along with iron, it is also required in the production of red blood cells.

- The crunchy, sweet yet delicate flavor of root lotus is because of its optimum electrolyte balance. While sodium gives the sweet taste to the root, potassium acts to counter negative effects of sodium by regulating heart rate and blood pressure.

Selection and storage:

Lotus root (renkon) harvest begins by August and last until fall. Traditionally, farmers sink knee-deep ponds and feel for the rhizome using their toes, which are then dug out by hand. Southeastern region of China and Lake Kasumigaura in Ibaraki prefecture in Japan is known for renkon production.

From the distance, lotus rhizomes appear as big size bananas arranged in sausage pattern. While buying, look for clean, firm roots with smooth unblemished skin. Fresh roots are readily available year-round in major cities in the US. One can also buy sliced, canned, and freeze-dried roots in the supermarkets or Japanese or other Asian stores.

Once at home, place the roots in cool, dark place away from humidity for 3-4 days. Uncut rhizomes can stay fresh for up to 2 weeks in the refrigerator.

Preparation:

Lotus root known as renkon in Japan and Lián ǒu in China has occupied a special place since centuries in their culture. The roots as well as seeds, raw or cooked, have found application in variety of oriental recipes in East, Southeast Asian, and Pacific regions.

To prepare, break the root at nodal intersections into individual parts. Wash the root thoroughly in cold running water before use. Trim the ends. Peel its inedible outer tough skin using paring knife to expose ice-white, daikon (radish) like flesh. It can be cut into cubes, or chopped to fine sticks in a ways desired like in other vegetables. Rinse the slices immediately in the vinegar or acidulated (lemon) water to prevent from discoloration.

Young, clean and tender rhizomes can be added raw in salads. However, mature rhizome taste bitter and can be eaten after cooking.

Renkon is one of the root vegetables used in tempura and kinpira style cooking.

Lotus root chips are popular snacks in Japan.

The root in India is featured in variety of curry, stews, and stir-fries.

Chinese use the root in soups, stuffing, stir-fries, etc.

In China, lotus seeds are eaten as snack.

A GROUP OF STARCHY VEGETABLES ALSO CONTAINING SUGAR

Photos can be found at:
http://vegetables.healthyfoodseries.com/starchy-vegetables/

Jicama
Sweet Potatoes
Squash, Winter
Yams
Pumpkins

JICAMA

Jicama, also known as yam bean, is a round, fleshy taproot vegetable of bean family plant. Its underground starchy root is one of the popular edible root vegetables grown in many parts of Central American, South Asian, Caribbean, and some Andean South American regions. It's refreshing; crispy, ice-white fruit-like pulp can be eaten raw or cooked in a variety of sweet and savory dishes worldwide.

Health Benefits:
- Jicama is very low calorie root vegetables. However, its high quality phyto-nutrition profile comprises of dietary fiber, and anti-oxidants, in

addition to small proportions of minerals, and vitamins.

- It is one of the finest source dietary fiber and excellent source of oligofructose inulin, a soluble dietary fiber. Inulin is a zero calorie, sweet inert carbohydrate and does not metabolize in the human body, which make the root an ideal sweet snack for diabetics and dieters.
- The tubers are rich in vitamin C. Vitamin-C is a powerful water-soluble anti-oxidant that helps body scavenge harmful free radicals, thereby offers protection from cancers, inflammation and viral cough and cold.
- It also contains small levels of some of valuable B-complex group of vitamins such as folates, riboflavin, pyridoxine, pantothenic acid and thiamin.
- Further, it provides healthy amounts of some important minerals like magnesium, copper, iron and manganese.

Selection and storage:

Jicamas are generally available year around in the markets. Generally, they enter through land route and flood the USA markets from the Central American countries during spring and summer.

Choose well-formed, firm, round, medium sized tubers. Avoid soft, shriveled, or tubers with surface cuts, cracks and bruise skin.

Once at home, jicamas can be stored much alike potatoes. They have very good shelf life and keep well in a cool, dry, dark place for about 3-4 weeks. Exposure to temperature below 10 °C results in chill-induced changes in color and texture. In addition, prolong storage converts starch to sugar, which makes the roots less sought after in savory dishes.

Cut sections, cubes or slices, however, should be placed inside the refrigerator.

Preparation:
Wash in cool running water and dry mop like in other tubers. Peel off thick fibrous skin using a vegetable peeler or paring knife. Peel and other plant parts contain *rotenene*, an organic poison; and therefore, should be discarded. It then can be cut into cubes, sliced, or chopped to fine sticks in a ways desired. It then can be cut into cubes, sliced, or chopped to fine sticks in a ways desired.

Fresh jicama is used much like a vegetable and is an important starch source in much of Central America. It stays crisp when cooked, making it one of the wonderful vegetable in stir-fries.

Raw jicama has sweet succulent apple like fruity taste. In many parts of Mexico, fresh tubers are cut into cubes/sticks and sprinkled with lime juice, salt and olive oil and paprika or ground chili pepper.

Jicama is a favorite root vegetable in Mexican cooking where it is used in salads, slaws, stews, stir-fries, soups, etc. with other common vegetables and fruits like orange, pineapple, carrot, green beans as well as with poultry, meat and seafood.

Outside of the American continent, this tuber is among the popular starch root in many south and southeast regions. Fresh young tubers are sliced and eaten with other fruits like pineapple, apple, raw mango, sweet potato, etc.

SWEET POTATO
(*Ipomoa Batatas*, Lamarck)

Sweet potato belongs to the morning-glory family. The edible portion is a swollen side root, not so nutritious or easily digested as the common white potato, and in composition differs from it in containing more sugar, gum, dextrin, pectose, and less starch.

Sweet potatoes should not be confused with yams, another starchy root commonly grown in Western Africa.

Sweet potatoes contain less starch and more sugar than whites. They must be cooked in a rather more careful manner. They should be mealy and tender when done, not heavy and sodden.

Orange-fleshed sweet potatoes may be one of nature's unsurpassed sources of beta-carotene. Several recent studies have shown the superior ability of sweet potatoes to raise our blood levels of vitamin A. This benefit may be particularly true for children. In several studies from Africa, sweet potatoes were found to contain between 100-1,600 micrograms (RAE) of vitamin A in every 3.5 ounces—enough, on average, to meet 35% of all vitamin A needs, and in many cases enough to meet over 90% of vitamin A needs (from this single food alone).

Sweet potatoes are not always orange-fleshed on the inside but can also be a spectacular purple color. Sometimes it's impossible to tell from the skin of sweet potato just how rich in purple tones its inside will be. The purple-fleshed sweet potato *anthocyanins*—primarily *peonidins* and *cyanidins*—have important antioxidant properties and anti-inflammatory properties. Particularly when passing through our digestive tract, they may be able to lower the potential health risk posed by heavy metals and oxygen radicals.

COMPOSITION

Water	.75.0
Albuminoids, etc	. 1.5
Starch	.15.0
Sugar	. 1.7
Dextrin, and gum	. 2.2
Pectose	. 0.9
Fat	. 0.4
Cellulose	. 1.8
Mineral matter	. 1.5

All varieties of sweet potatoes may be cooked after the same rules. Containing sugar as well as starch, they are easily made pasty or heavy by careless cooking and under such conditions are dense and difficult of digestion. Cooked with fat they are much more objectionable than white potatoes under the same conditions.

Health Benefits:

- Sweet potato, not only is just sweet to your taste buds but also good for your cardiovascular health.
- Sweet potato is one of the average calorie starch foods. The tuber, however, contains no saturated fats or cholesterol and is rich source of dietary fiber, anti-oxidants, vitamins, and minerals.
- Its calorie content mainly comes from starch, a complex carbohydrate. Sweet potato has higher amylose to the amylopectin ratio than potato. Amylose raises the blood sugar levels *slowly* on comparison to simple sugars and therefore, recommended as a healthy food supplement even in diabetes.
- The tuber is an excellent source of *flavonoid phenolic compounds* such as beta-carotene and vitamin A. The value is one of the highest among the root-vegetables categories. These compounds are powerful natural antioxidants. Vitamin A is also required by the body to maintain integrity of healthy mucus membranes and skin. It is a vital nutrient for acuity of vision. Consumption of natural vegetables and fruits rich in flavonoids helps to protect from lung and oral cavity cancers.

- The tubers are packed with many essential vitamins such as pantothenic acid (vitamin B-5), pyridoxine(vitamin B-6), and thiamin (vitamin B-1), niacin, and riboflavin. These vitamins are essential in the sense that body requires them from external sources to replenish. These vitamins function as co-factors for various enzymes during metabolism.
- Sweet potato provides a good amount of vital minerals such as iron, calcium, magnesium, manganese, and potassium that are very essential for enzyme, protein, and carbohydrate metabolism.
- Sweet potato leaves are indeed more nutritious than the tuber itself. Fresh leaves contain more iron, vitamin C, folates, vitamin K, and potassium but less sodium than the tuber.

Selection and storage:

Although sweet potato leaves are being eaten in some parts of the world, the root that is the toast of sweet potato lovers. In the store, buy fresh tubers with intact smooth skin and firm to woody consistency. Go for organic varieties for best taste and nutrition levels.

Avoid soft, flabby, or wilted roots. As in potatoes, sprouting would make them lose flavor and less desirable.

Wash them in clean running water to remove sand and soil. They should be stored in a cool, dark, and well-ventilated place.

Preparation:

To prepare, wash the root in cold water. It can be eaten raw with skin. However, for baking preparations, its skin may be peeled off before or after cooked.

Some serving ideas:

- Fresh sweet potatoes can be eaten raw.
- Baking in water with a pinch of salt would gives them a rich taste. Peel the skin before eating.
- Camote, sweet potato known in the Latin world, is used extensively in the Mexican cuisine.
- *Camote cue*, where in the tuber deep-fried and caramelized with brown sugar, is a popular street food in the Philippines.
- It sweet flesh used in soups, curries, stews, and in confectionary to make cakes, pie, etc.
- The tuber also used to prepare different kinds of baby foods.
- Sweet potato chips are enjoyed as favorite snacks.

Safety Precaution:

Sweet potatoes contain *oxalic acid,* a naturally occurring substance found in some vegetables that may crystallize as oxalate stones in the urinary tract in some people.

YAMS

Yams look and taste like sweet potatoes and may be cooked after the same rules. They do not, however, belong to the same order of plants. The common yam is *Dioscorea Alata*, but other species of the same genus are used. The Chinese yam *(Dioscorea Batatas)* is imported into the United States and used by many in place of our common sweet potatoes. They are exceedingly large, frequently weighing from two to four or six pounds. The so-called yam of the Southern United States is simply a larger variety of the common sweet potato.

Creamy or firm when cooked, yams have an earthy, hardy taste and usually a minimal amount of sweetness. Although they are available throughout the year their season runs from October through December when they are at their best.

There are approximately 200 different varieties of yams with flesh colors varying from white to ivory to yellow to purple while their thick skin comes in white, pink or brownish-black. Their shape is long and cylindrical (oftentimes having offshoots referred to as "toes") while their exterior texture is rough and scaly. There is great confusion between yams and sweet potatoes in the United States; most of the vegetables labeled "yams" in the markets are really orange-colored sweet potatoes.

COMPOSITION

```
Water . . . . . . . . . . . . . . . . .79.6
Albuminoids, etc. . . . . . . . . . . . 2.2
Carbohydrates . . . . . . . . . . . .15.3
Fat . . . . . . . . . . . . . . . . . 0.5
Cellulose . . . . . . . . . . . . . . 0.9
Mineral matter . . . . . . . . . . . . 1.5
```

Health Benefits:

- Yam is a good source of energy; 100 g provides 118 calories. It is mainly composed of complex carbohydrates and soluble dietary fiber. Together, they raise blood sugar levels rather slower than simple sugars and therefore, recommended as the low glycemic index healthy food. In addition, dietary fiber helps reduce constipation, decrease bad (LDL) cholesterol levels by binding to it in the intestines and prevent colon cancer risks by preventing toxic compounds in the food from adhering to the colon mucosa.

- The tuber is an excellent source of B-complex group of vitamins. It provides adequate daily requirements of pyridoxine (vitamin B6), thiamin (vitamin B1), riboflavin, folic acid, pantothenic acid and niacin. These vitamins mediate various metabolic functions in the body.

- Fresh root also contains good amounts of anti-oxidant vitamin; vitamin-C. Vitamin C has important roles in anti-aging, immune function, wound healing, bone growth.

- They contain small amounts of vitamin-A, and beta-carotene levels. Carotenes convert to vitamin A in the body. Both these compounds are strong antioxidants. Vitamin A has many functions like maintaining healthy mucus membranes and skin, night vision, growth and protection from lung and oral cavity cancers.
- Further, the tuber is indeed one of the vegetables rich sources of minerals like copper, calcium, potassium, iron, manganese, and phosphorus. Potassium is an important component of cell and body fluids, which helps controlling heart rate and blood pressure by countering hypertensive effects of sodium. Copper is required in the production of red blood cells. Manganese is used by the body as a co-factor for the antioxidant enzyme, *superoxide dismutase*. Iron is required for red blood cell formation.

Selection and storage:

Yams are available in the market year around. Fresh tubers, however, are more plentiful by August when the annual harvest season begins at the end of the rainy season in western Africa. A new yam festival celebrated in symbolism to fresh crop and availability of fresh food in abundance all over Nigeria and Ghana with great fervor.

49

In the super-markets generally you find small cut sections wrapped in thin plastic covers. Their interior meat is white to light pink depending up on the cultivar type with rich starchy flavor.

In general, whole tubers are stored after drying several hours in the sunlight, in well-ventilated yam barns (traditional storage system), where they stay well for several months without refrigeration. Cut sections, however, are used early or stored in the refrigerator for immediate use.

Preparation:

Unlike sweet potatoes, which can be eaten raw, yams should never be eaten uncooked since they contain many naturally-occurring plant toxins including dioscorin, diosgenin and tri-terpenes. They must be peeled and cooked in order to remove these bitter proteins.

Dioscorea opposita or Japanese yam is, however, eaten raw unlike its African brethren. Here, the whole tuber is briefly soaked in a vinegar-water solution to neutralize irritant oxalate crystals found in their skin. The root is then cut into small slices or grated to get a gel-like milk to add mouth-watering oriental recipes.

Some preparation ideas:
- The tuber can be used in variety of cuisines boiled, baked, fried, or sometimes roasted.
- The most common cooking method in Africa is "pounded yam." Fufu (Foo-foo, Foufou) is a special dish prepared during the yam festival. To

make fufu: either pounded yam or its powder is added to boiling water to make a cake like mass. A bite-sized piece of the fufu is torn from cake and consumed with sauce, stew, or soup akin to ragi cake (finger-millet, Eleusine coracana) eaten in some parts of south India.

- Japanese yam or *yamaimo* is eaten raw as salads or grated to get a gel-like milk, which is added to noodles.
- It is also used like sweet potatoes in the preparation of cake, casseroles, breads, etc.

Medical uses:

Yam tubers are used various traditional medicines in China, Korea and Japan. The mucilaginous tuber milk contains allantoin, a cell-proliferate that speeds the healing process when applied externally to ulcers, boils, and abscesses. Its decoction is also used to stimulate appetite and to relieve bronchial irritation, cough, etc.

Safety Precaution:

Yams of African species must be cooked before safely eaten, because various natural toxin substances such as dioscorine can cause illness if consumed raw.

WINTER SQUASH
(*Cucurbita maxima*, Duchesne)

Winter squash, members of the *Cucurbitaceae* family and relatives of both the melon and the cucumber, come in many different varieties. While each type varies in shape, color, size and flavor, they all share some common characteristics. Their shells are hard and difficult to pierce, enabling them to have long storage periods between one week and six months. Their flesh is mildly sweet in flavor and finely grained in texture. Additionally, all have seed-containing hollow inner cavities.

We are just beginning to discover the wealth of nourishment supplied by the mildly sweet flavored and finely textured winter squash, a vegetable that was once such an important part of the diet of the Native Americans that they buried it along with the dead to provide them nourishment on their final journey. Winter squash is available from August through March; however, they are at their best from October to November when they are in season.

Like other vegetables in this group, the winter squash is served in place of potatoes or rice; it is not, however, so rich in nourishment, but gives variety to the daily menu.

Butternut squash is the most popular winter squash variety. It is recognized as a large pear shaped golden-yellow pumpkin fruit.

Health Benefits:

- Butternut squash contains many vital poly-phenolic anti-oxidants and vitamins. It is rich source of dietary fiber and phyto-nutrients. Squash is one of the common vegetables that often recommended by dieticians in the cholesterol controlling and weight reduction programs.
- It has more vitamin A than that in pumpkin. Vitamin A is a powerful natural anti-oxidant and is required by the body for maintaining the integrity of skin and mucus membranes. It is also an essential vitamin for good eye-sight. Research studies suggest that natural foods rich in vitamin A help the body protected against lung and oral cavity cancers.
- Furthermore, butternut squash has plenty of natural poly-phenolic flavonoid compounds like α and β-carotenes, cryptoxanthin-β, and lutein. These compounds convert to vitamin A inside the body and deliver same protective functions of vitamin A on the body.
- It is rich in B-complex group of vitamins like folates, riboflavin, niacin, vitamin B-6 (pyridoxine), thiamin, and pantothenic acid.
- It has similar mineral profile as that in pumpkin, containing adequate levels of minerals like iron, zinc, copper, calcium, potassium, and phosphorus.
- Butternut squash seeds are a good source of dietary fiber and mono-unsaturated fatty acids that benefit for heart health. In addition, they are rich in protein, minerals, and numerous health-benefiting vitamins. The seeds are an excellent source of health promoting

amino acid, tryptophan. Tryptophan converts to health benefiting GABA neuro-chemical in the brain.

Selection and storage:

Being a winter-squash member, butternuts are readily available in the USA markets from September until the middle of December. However, since many fruits arrive from South American continent, they can be easily found all around the season.

Buy well-grown whole butternut squash instead of its sections. Look for mature product that features fine woody note on tapping, and heavy in hand. Its stem should be stout and firmly attached to the fruit.

Avoid those with wrinkled surface, spots, cuts, and bruises.

Once at home, well-ripen squash can be stored for many weeks in cool, humid-free, well-ventilated place at room temperature. However, cut sections should be placed inside the refrigerator where they keep well for few days.

Preparation:

As in pumpkins, some hybrid squash varieties are generally subjected to insecticide powder or spray. Therefore, wash them thoroughly in running water in order to remove dust, soil and any residual insecticides/fungicides.

Whenever possible, buy long neck butternut fruit as it contains more meat and fewer hollow cavities and seeds. Cut the stem end and slice the whole fruit into two equal halves. Remove central net-like structure and set aside seeds. Then cut into desired sizes. In general, wedges/small cubes are used in cooking preparations.

Almost all the parts of the butternut squash plant; fruit, leaves, flowers, and seeds are edible.

Butternut squash has a nutty flavor and mildly sweet taste. Fresh raw cubes may be added to vegetable salads.

The squash adds flavor to both savory and sweet dishes.

It can be baked, stuffed, stew-fried; however, steam cooking gives the maximum nutrients.

Roasted and tossed butternut squash seeds can be used as snacks.

PUMPKIN
(*Cucurbita Pepo*, Linn.)

Pumpkin squash is a fruit that belongs to the gourd family. The fruit has a round shape but appears to be flattened at the top and bottom. It may also have an oblong shape. The weight of the fruit ranges from 1 pound to several hundred pounds. Smaller pumpkins known as the sugar or pie pumpkin are the sweetest. The pumpkin has a thick outer shell that is orange or deep yellow in color. However, some varieties may be green, red or gray in color. The interior has a deep orange color. Plenty of edible seeds known as pepitas are found inside the fruit. It has high amounts of vitamins A and C. It also contains vitamins B1, B3, B5 and B6. Mineral content includes potassium, magnesium, iron, calcium, copper and phosphorous. The fruit can also help you meet your dietary fiber requirements.

Health Benefits:

- It is one of the very low calorie vegetables and contains no saturated fats or cholesterol; however, it is rich in dietary fiber, anti-oxidants, minerals, vitamins. The vegetable is one of the food items recommended by dieticians in cholesterol controlling and weight reduction programs.

- Pumpkin is a storehouse of many anti-oxidant vitamins such as vitamin-A, vitamin-C and vitamin-E.

- It is high in vitamin-A. Vitamin A is a powerful natural anti-oxidant and is required by the body for maintaining the integrity of skin and mucus membranes. It is also an essential vitamin for good visual sight. Research studies suggest that natural foods rich in vitamin A help a body protects against lung and oral cavity cancers.

- It is also an excellent source of many natural poly-phenolic flavonoid compounds such as α, ß carotenes, cryptoxanthin, lutein and zea-xanthin. Carotenes convert into vitamin A inside the body.

- Zea-xanthin is a natural anti-oxidant which has UV (ultra-violet) rays filtering actions in the macula lutea in retina of the eyes. Thus, it helps protect from "age-related macular disease" (ARMD) in the elderly.

- The fruit is a good source of B-complex group of vitamins like folates, niacin, vitamin B-6 (pyridoxine), thiamin and pantothenic acid.
- It is also rich source of minerals like copper, calcium, potassium and phosphorus.
- Pumpkin seeds indeed are an excellent source of dietary fiber and mono-unsaturated fatty acids, which are good for heart health. In addition, the seeds are concentrated sources of protein, minerals and health-benefiting vitamins. Further, the seeds are an excellent source of health promoting amino acid tryptophan. Tryptophan is converted to GABA in the brain.

Selection and storage:

Pumpkins are readily available in the market year around. Buy well grown whole pumpkin instead of sections. Look for mature product that features fine woody note on tapping, heavy in hand and dry, stout stem. Avoid the one with wrinkled surface, cuts and bruises.

Once at home, fully ripen pumpkin can be stored for many weeks at cool, well-ventilated place at room temperature. However, cut sections should be placed inside the refrigerator where it can keep well for a few days.

Preparation:

Some hybrid varieties are usually subjected to insecticide powder or spray. Therefore, wash them thoroughly in running water in order to remove dust, soil and any residual insecticides/fungicides.

Cut the stem end and slice the whole fruit into two equal halves. Remove central net like structure and set aside seeds. Then cut into desired sizes. In general, small cubes are used in cooking preparations.

Almost all the parts of the pumpkin plant; fruit, leaves, flowers and seeds, are edible.

Pumpkin can be used in a variety of delicious recipes either baked, stew-fried; however, eaten best by steam cooking in order to get maximum nutrients.

In China, the leaves of this plant are consumed as cooked greens or in soups.

In the Indian subcontinent it is popular in sweet dishes, desserts, soups, curries, etc.

The fruit is used in the preparation of pies, pancakes, custard, ravioli, etc.

Golden nugget pumpkins are used to make soufflés, stuffing, soups, etc.

Roasted Pumpkin seeds can be eaten as snacks.

A GROUP OF SUCCULENT VEGETABLES CONTAINING A LITTLE STARCH AND SUGAR

Photos found at: http://vegetables.healthyfoodseries.com/succulent-vege...arch-and-sugar/

Salsify
Parsnips
String Beans

In this group will be found succulent vegetables containing about an equal amount of starch and sugar; not enough, however, to take the place of rice or potato, but sufficient to make them objectionable to diabetic persons. They are not valuable nutrients, and are placed among succulent vegetables as containing mineral matter and the necessary bulk.

SALSIFY

Salsify or oyster plant (*Tragopogon porrifolius,* Linn.) is an edible root resembling a small parsnip, and may be cooked and served according to the same rules. Owing to a peculiar fishy flavor it is frequently called vegetable oyster, and is used by vegetarians in imitation of the real oyster. It makes a delicious mock oyster soup; a recipe for which will be found under soups.

PARSNIPS

Parsnip is the root of the *Pastinaca sativa*, Linn. It resembles the carrot in general appearance, except that it is white, and contains both sugar and starch. Being rich in woody fibre, the parsnip must be carefully cooked to be palatable and wholesome; they are usually served as an accompaniment to salt fish. Its long tuberous root has cream-colored skin and flesh and can be left in the ground when mature as it becomes sweeter in flavour after winter frosts.

The parsnip is native to Eurasia. It has been used as a vegetable since ancient times and was cultivated by the Romans, although there is some confusion in the literature of the time between parsnips and carrots. It was used as a sweetener before the arrival in Europe of cane sugar. It was introduced into the United States in the nineteenth century.

COMPOSITION OF THE PARSNIP

Water	.82.0
Albuminoids, etc.	1.2
Sugar	5.0
Starch	3.5
Pectose, dextrin, etc.	3.7
Fat	1.5
Cellulose	2.1
Mineral matter	1.0

Parsnips are digested principally in the intestines.

Health Benefits:

- Generally, parsnip contains more sugar than carrots, radish,_turnips. Nonetheless, its sweet, juicy root is rich in several health-benefiting phyto-nutrients, vitamins, minerals, and fiber.
- It is one of the excellent sources of soluble and insoluble dietary fiber. Adequate fiber in the diet helps reduce blood cholesterol levels, obesity and constipation conditions.
- As in carrots and other members of apiaceae family vegetables, parsnip too contains many poly-acetylene anti-oxidants such as *falcarinol, falcarindiol, panaxydiol,* and *methyl-falcarindiol.*
- Several research studies from scientists at University of Newcastle at Tyne found that these compounds have anti-inflammatory, anti-fungal, and anti-cancer function and offer protection from colon cancer and acute lymphoblastic leukemia (ALL).
- Fresh roots are also good in vitamin C. Vitamin C is a powerful water-soluble anti-oxidant, easily available to us from natural sources. It helps the body maintain healthy connective tissue, teeth, and gum. Its anti-oxidant property helps protect from diseases and cancers by scavenging harmful free radicals from the body.

- Further, the root is rich in many B-complex groups of vitamins such as folic acid, vitamin B-6 (pyridoxine), thiamin, and pantothenic acid as well as vitamin K and vitamin E.
- In addition, it also has healthy levels of minerals like iron, calcium, copper, potassium, manganese and phosphorus. Potassium is an important component of cell and body fluids that helps controlling heart rate and blood pressure by countering effects of sodium.

Selection and storage:

Parsnip season begins soon after the first frost and last until March. It is not uncommon to find parsnips and carrots grown by many families in their home garden during the season.

In the markets select fresh, firm, fleshy, medium size, even surfaced parsnips. Avoid long, thin, and tail like roots, as they are stringy and less sought after in cooking. Furthermore, avoid, woody, over-mature ones, as they are off-flavored. Do not buy soft, shriveled, pitted, knobby, or damaged roots.

Store parsnips in a plastic bag and place in the vegetable drawer of the refrigerator. Do not place raw parsnips in the freezer compartment.

Preparation:

To prepare, wash them in cold water and scrub or gently peel the skin. Trim off the ends. Cut into cubes, disc, and pieces as you desire.

Tender parsnips cooked in a similar way like carrots. Do not overcook; indeed, they cook early as they contain more sugar than starch.

Raw parsnips add unique sweet taste to salads, coleslaw, and toppings.

It can be cooked and massed with potato, leeks, cauliflower, etc.

Slices and cubes can be added to stews, soups, and stir-fries.

It can be used in breads, pies, casseroles, cakes, etc.

STRING BEANS
(*Haricots Verts*)

COMPOSITION

Water 89.5
Proteids 1.5
Carbo-hydrates 7.3
Fat 0.4
Cellulose 0.6
Mineral matter 0.7

Because of their rich green color, we don't always think about green beans as providing us with important amounts of colorful pigments like carotenoids. But they do! Recent studies have confirmed the presence of lutein, beta-carotene, violaxanthin, and neoxanthin in green beans. In some cases, the presence of these carotenoids in green beans is comparable to their presence in other carotenoid-rich vegetables like carrots and tomatoes. The only reason we don't see these carotenoids is because of the concentrated chlorophyll content of green beans and the amazing shades of green that it provides.

If you are unable to obtain fresh green beans, you can still get many valuable nutrients from green beans that have been frozen or canned. We like fresh greens the best! But we realize that access to them can sometimes be a problem. When first frozen and then cooked, retention of some B vitamins in green beans (like vitamins B6 and B2) can be as high as 90%. Recent studies have shown that canned green beans, on average, lose about one third of their phenolic compounds during the canning process. They lose B vitamins as well but in the case of some B vitamins like folic acid, as little as 10%.

Green beans (referred to as "string beans" by the study authors) have recently been shown to have impressive antioxidant capacity. Research comparing the overall antioxidant capacity of green beans to other foods in the pea and bean families (for example, snow peas or winged beans) has found green beans to come out on top, even though green beans are not always highest in their concentration of specific antioxidant nutrients like phenolic acids or vitamin C. It's not surprising to find recent studies highlighting the antioxidant capacity of green beans!

They contain sufficient starch and sugar, however, to be detrimental to diabetic persons. To be easily digested and palatable they must be used fresh and while the pod is young and tender. String beans are waste or bulk food and are principally digested in the intestines.

Health Benefits:
- Fresh green beans are very low in calories and contain no saturated fat. Nevertheless, the lean vegetables are a very good source of vitamins, minerals, and plant derived micronutrients.
- They are very rich source of dietary fiber which acts as a bulk laxative that helps to protect the mucous membrane of the colon by decreasing its exposure time to toxic substances as well as by binding to cancer-causing chemicals in the colon. Adequate amount of fiber has also been shown to reduce blood cholesterol levels by decreasing reabsorption of cholesterol-binding bile acids in the colon.
- Green beans contain excellent levels of vitamin A, and health promoting flavonoid poly phenolic antioxidants such as lutein, zea-xanthin and ß-carotene in good amounts. These compounds help act as protective scavengers against oxygen-derived free radicals and reactive oxygen species (ROS) that play a role in aging and various disease processes.

- Zea-xanthin, an important dietary carotenoid in the beans, selectively absorbed into the retinal macula lutea in the eyes where it thought to provide antioxidant and protective UV light filtering functions. It is, therefore, green beans offer some protection in preventing *age-related macular disease* (ARMD) in the elderly.

- Snap beans are a good source of *folates.* Folate along with vitamin B-12 is one of the essential components of DNA synthesis and cell division. Good folate diet when given during preconception periods and during pregnancy helps prevent neural-tube defects among the offspring.

- They also contain good amounts of vitamin-B6 (pyridoxine), thiamin (vitamin B-1), and vitamin-C. Consumption of foods rich in vitamin C helps the body develop resistance against infectious agents and scavenge harmful oxygen-free radicals.

- In addition, beans contain healthy amounts of minerals like iron, calcium, magnesium, manganese, and potassium, which are very essential for body metabolism. Manganese is a co-factor for the antioxidant enzyme, *superoxide dismutase,* which is a very powerful free radical scavenger. Potassium is an important component of cell and body fluids that helps controlling heart rate and blood pressure.

66

Selection and storage:

Raw fresh green beans, also called as *snap beans* or *French beans*, should be tender, long, stiff, but flexible and give snap sound when broken. Buy them from organic stores for their rich "beany" flavor.

Avoid limp or overly matured beans with tough skin.

To store, place them in a perforated plastic bag and keep inside the refrigerator set at high relative humidity. They keep well for up to a week.

Preparation:

Wash raw beans in cold water. Just before using, remove the strings and trim the ends.

Green beans are among the most-favored vegetable items in stir-fry, stews, grilled-salads, steamed along with carrots, cauliflower, peas, tomato...etc.

They mix well with cheese, nuts, mushroom, seafood, meat, etc.

In Asian region, they are used in curries, soups, stir-fry with rice, etc.

A GROUP OF VEGETABLES CONTAINING NITROGEN AND STARCH

Photos found at: http://vegetables.healthyfoodseries.com/vegetables-containing-nitrogen-and-starch-2/

> Old dried peas
> Lentils
> Old dried beans of all varieties
> Chick peas
> Ground or peanuts

To this same family belong clover, alfalfa, cow pea, and many other plants of economic importance. This group contains edible leguminous seeds, characterized by the large amount of nitrogenous matter they contain. As flesh formers or muscle and tissue building foods, they far excel the seeds of the cereal grasses. The amount of nitrogen in dry beans is double that in mature wheat. The albuminoids are present in a substance known as legumin, a vegetable casein. The Chinese take advantage of this peculiar form of nitrogen, and by certain methods make the pulp of both old peas and beans into a cheese which very closely resembles that made from cows' milk. These vegetables, being rich in nitrogen, should be used in the place of meat, not with meat, and should be served with foods containing non-nitrogenous or carbonaceous nutrients; for instance, fat pork and beans, rice and lentils, dried peas and bacon are samples of the best form of blending.

Legumin is digested and absorbed at a slower rate than the albuminoids of milk, eggs and meat; hence, these vegetables are unfit for daily food for persons whose occupation confines them in close and ill-ventilated rooms, or where little exercise can be taken. They are exceedingly valuable for the outdoor laborer; being less in price they may be substituted frequently for meat.

PEAS

Peas (*Pisum sativum*, Linn.) are the seeds of a leguminous plant. When mature and ripe (old and dried) they contain according to Payne

Nitrogenous matter 23.8
Starch, etc. 58.7
Cellulose 3.5
Fatty matter 2. 1
Mineral matter 2. 1
Water 8.3

Although they belong to the same family as beans and lentils, they are usually distinguished as a separate group because of the ways in which they are prepared. The different types of peas are all spherical, a feature that also sets them apart from beans and lentils. Dried peas are produced by harvesting the peapods when they are fully mature and then

69

drying them. Once they are dried and the skins removed, they split naturally.

Dried peas, a small but nutritionally mighty member of the legume family, are a very good source of cholesterol-lowering fiber. Not only can dried peas help lower cholesterol, they are also of special benefit in managing blood-sugar disorders since their high fiber content prevents blood sugar levels from rising rapidly after a meal.

Fiber is far from all that dried peas have to offer. Dried peas also provide good to excellent amounts of four important minerals, two B-vitamins, and protein--all with virtually no fat. As if this weren't enough, dried peas also feature isoflavones (notably *daidzein*). Isoflavones are phytonutrients that can act like weak estrogens in the body and whose dietary consumption has been linked to a reduced risk of certain health conditions, including breast and prostate cancer.

Nitrogenous foods are principally digested in the stomach and are muscle and tissue builders. Peas contain starch and fat, both carbonaceous elements. Starches are digested in the small intestines and fats are emulsionized. While peas contain nitrogenous matter and starch, the starch is insufficient to make a balanced ration. Serve with them fat, as bacon, or other starchy food, as potatoes or rice. Served with fat and starch, as white bread and butter, they form a typical food, and one would have in this combination a highly nutritious diet. It is estimated by Hutchinson that a level tablespoonful of peameal made into a plate of thick water soup will have the proteid value of one ounce of meat.

If milk mstead of water is used, the proteid would be at least double. Old or dried peas must be soaked over night that they may take up the same amount of water with which they parted in the drying. This reduces their nutritive value from the table given.

The field pea (*Pisum arvense*, Linn.), sometimes called the commercial pea, is not used in this country as food for man.

The chick pea (*Cicer arietinum*, Linn.) is not commonly known to American people; it can be purchased, however, in some of the Jewish markets of New York. It is highly nitrogenous, and is said to be the pulse referred to in the Bible. It is usually toasted and eaten the same as peanuts. It is used in small quantities in Spain and extensively in the East. The Arabs when crossing the desert carry chick peas, feeling that they have with them a typical or perfect food.

Split peas are dried peas with the tough envelope removed, which allows them to divide easily into halves; they are much more easily cooked than those dried in the husk or skin.

Young or green peas served as succulent vegetables, not rich in nitrogen, are considered under vegetables containing sugar.

GREEN PEAS

Peas, like corn, lose their sweetness very quickly after picking. Fresh peas should not be shelled until just before the time of cooking; then wash them quickly in cold water, drain, throw into a kettle of boiling water, add a teaspoonful of salt to harden the water. This will prevent the skins from cracking. Boil rapidly from ten to twenty minutes. After they have been boiling ten minutes, take out one or two and press with a fork; if they mash easily they are done. Drain, turn into a hot dish, add a lump of butter the size of a walnut, and serve.

The most important point in cooking peas is to have plenty of water. The water must be slightly salted and the peas boiled just long enough to become tender, and drained at once. In this way they will retain their color and sweetness. There are many varieties of pests, many of which are coarse and only fit for drying. The choice kinds of garden peas are, of course, sweet, nutritious and wholesome. There is also a kind of pea called sugar pea, the pods of which are gathered young and cooked and eaten with the seeds in, the same way as we use string beans. Boiled, and dressed with butter, salt and pepper, they are delicious.

If peas are old or have been picked some time before cooking, it is very difficult to make them tender. Indeed, the longer they are boiled, the harder they become. In this condition they are not digestible. It is best to save them for another meal, and by pressing them through a sieve they may be made into a palatable and digestible soup.

Health Benefits:
- Green peas are one of the most nutritious leguminous vegetables, rich in health benefiting phyto-nutrients, minerals, vitamins and anti-oxidants.

- Peas are relatively low in calories on comparison with beans, and cowpeas. Nonetheless, the legumes are a good source of proteins, and soluble as well as insoluble fiber.
- Fresh pea pods are excellent source of folic acid. Folates are B-complex vitamins required for DNA synthesis inside the cell. Well established research studies suggest that adequate folate rich foods in expectant mothers would help prevent neural tube defects in the newborn babies.
- Fresh green peas are very good in ascorbic acid (vitamin C). Vitamin C is a powerful natural water-soluble anti-oxidant. Vegetables rich in this vitamin helps body develop resistance against infectious agents and scavenge harmful, pro-inflammatory free radicals from the body.
- Peas contain phytosterols especially ß-sitosterol. Studies suggest that vegetables like legumes, fruits and cereals rich in plant sterols help lower cholesterol levels in the body.
- Garden peas are also good in vitamin K. Vitamin K has found to have a potential role in bone mass building function by promoting osteo-trophic activity in the bone. It also has established role in Alzheimer's disease patients by limiting neuronal damage in the brain.
- Fresh green peas also contain adequate amounts of anti-oxidants flavonoids such as carotenes, lutein and zea-xanthin as well as vitamin-A.

Vitamin A is an essential nutrient required for maintaining health of mucus membranes, skin and eye-sight. Further, consumption of natural fruits rich in flavonoids helps to protect from lung and oral cavity cancers.

- In addition to folates, peas are also good in many other essential B-complex vitamins such as pantothenic acid, niacin, thiamin, and pyridoxine. Furthermore, they are rich source of many minerals such as calcium, iron, copper, zinc, and manganese.

Selection and storage:

Green peas are winter crops. Fresh peas are readily sold from December until April in the market. However, dry, mature seeds, and split peas, flour...etc., are made available in the markets year round.

While shopping for green peas look for fresh pods that are full, heavy in hands and brimming with seeds. Avoid those with wrinkled surface or over-matured, yellow colored pods.

Green-peas are at their best soon after their harvest since much of sugar content in the seeds rapidly converts to starch. If you have to store at all, place them in the vegetable compartment inside the home refrigerator, set with high relative humidity where they keep fresh for 2-3 days. Frozen seeds can be used for several months.

Preparation:

Trim away the stalk and thin fiber along the suture line. Split open the outer coat to release round to oval, green seeds.

Peas mix well with other complementing vegetables like potato, carrot, beets, onion, artichokes, etc.

Pea soup is a flavorful side-dish.

BEANS
KIDNEY BEANS

(*Phaseolus vulgaris*, Linn.)

This one variety covers nearly all the beans in common use as food for man. The common soup or kidney bean, the Boston white beans used for baking, and the red bean may all be cooked in precisely the same manner. Haricots are small white beans. While the different varieties give just a trifle more or less nitrogenous matter, one analysis will serve for the whole.

The broad or Windsor bean (*Faba vulgaris*, Moench) is said to contain more nitrogen than other varieties.

COMPOSITION OF HARICOT BEANS

Water 14.0
Albuminoids, etc. 23.0
Starch, etc. 52.3

Fat 2.3
Cellulose 5.5
Mineral matter 2.9

All beans as butter, kidney, caseknife and flageolets may be cooked in precisely the same manner. The main points to be remembered are that all dried beans must be soaked overnight in cold water, and cooked in soft, unsalted water just at or below the boiling point, not boiled rapidly. Water rapidly boiled is precisely the same in temperature as that boiled slowly, but the motion of the water washes off the outside of the beans and destroys their texture.

LIMA BEANS

(*Phaseolus lunatus*, Linn.)

These beans are both "climbers" and "bush." They are characterized by being flat and larger than the ordinary kidney bean, and contain a trifle more starch and less nitrogen. As the hull of beans is indigestible, it is always wise to blanch and remove, or "pulp" them. Cook carefully that they may become soft without falling apart.

BLACK OR TURTLE BEANS

(*Dolichos Lablab*, Linn.)

On account of the black coloring matter contained in these seeds, they are used principally for mock turtle soup, or what is commonly known as black bean soup. They are, however, excellent when well cooked, pressed through a colander, and served in puree.

RED BEANS

The red Mexican beans are simply a variety of kidney bean. The flesh of the bean is perfectly white; the outside skin is red, and during the cooking colors the centre of the bean. With tomato and chilli sauce these make an admirable dinner dish and take the place of meat. Macaroni or spaghetti are usually served with them.

SOY BEAN (*Glycine hispida*, Maxim.)

Soy beans are grown principally in China where they form an important article of food; in fact, they are the richest of all in food constituents. It is also grown to a considerable extent in India, where it is mixed with rice. This bean ranks high in fat and albuminoids and is their only muscle-making food. It has more than meat value. By the Chinese it is made into cheese, pastes and sauces. Soy sauce is used by them on all meat and fish dishes. For the English and Americans it forms the foundation for such sauces as club-house and Worcestershire. Soy is an agreeable seasoning to creamed meat dishes and a very pleasant addition to French salad dressing. It can be purchased in jugs at any Chinese shop, or at the American wholesale druggists by measure.

Albuminoids, etc.	35.3
Fat	18.9
Starch and Dextrin	12.5
Sugar	12.0
Cellulose	4.2
Water	12.5
Mineral Matter	4.6

LENTILS

(*Lens esculenta*, Moench)

These are one of the most important of the leguminous seeds and are valuable for soups, stews and rice dishes in which there is a small allowance of nitrogenous elements.

Lentils are legumes along with other types of beans. They grow in pods that contain either one or two lentil seeds that are round, oval or heart-shaped disks and are oftentimes smaller than the tip of a pencil eraser. They may be sold whole or split into halves with the brown and green varieties being the best at retaining their shape after cooking.

Compared to other types of dried beans, lentils are relatively quick and easy to prepare. They readily absorb a variety of wonderful flavors from other foods and seasonings, are high in nutritional value and are available throughout the year.

Lentils, a small but nutritionally mighty member of the legume family, are a very good source of cholesterol-lowering fiber. Not only do lentils help lower cholesterol, they are of special benefit in managing blood-sugar disorders since their high fiber content prevents blood sugar levels from rising rapidly after a meal. But this is far from all lentils have to offer. Lentils also provide good to excellent amounts of six important minerals, two B-vitamins, and protein—all with virtually no fat. The calorie cost of all this nutrition? Just 230 calories for a whole cup of cooked lentils. This tiny nutritional giant fills you up—not out.

Wash and soak a pint of lentils overnight, in the morning drain, cover with warm, soft water and bring quickly to a boiling point. Boil gently about one hour, drain and cover again with fresh, boiling, soft water. Boil gently until the lentils are tender, about another hour. Press them between the thumb and fingers, if they mash quickly under pressure they are done. Drain in a colander. Put two tablespoonfuls of butter in a saucepan, when melted add the lentils; add one tablespoonful of onion juice, a palatable seasoning of salt and pepper; stir over the fire about fifteen minutes and serve very hot. One or two tablespoonfuls of cream may also be added if liked.

While the nitrogenous matter in lentils is greater than that in peas and beans, it is presented in a more digestible form. There is no doubt that lentils are the best and most easily digested of nitrogenous vegetables; they take the place of lean meats and should be served with rice, potatoes or other starchy foods.

COMPOSITION OF HUSKED LENTILS

```
Water . . . . . . . . . . . . . . . .12.5
Albuminoids . . . . . . . . . . . .25.0
Starch . . . . . . . . . . . . . . . .56.1
Fat . . . . . . . . . . . . . . . . . . 2.0
Cellulose . . . . . . . . . . . . . . 1.9
Mineral Matter . . . . . . . . . . . 2.5
```

The red, or Arabian lentils, are rich in iron, rarely ever come to this country, and when they do, only in small quantities, and sell at a high price. The *Revelenta arabica*, sold at a dollar a pound, is red lentil flour, used principally with milk for making soup or gruel for nursing mothers; it is said to produce milk of excellent quality. It is also used in purees or souffles in cases of neurasthenia.

Lentils should be served in every household at least once a week. They form an excellent substitute for flesh. In appearance they resemble a dark, tiny split pea; they are round but flat, not globular, like peas. While extensively grown in the United States they are principally used by the Germans.

CHICK PEAS

Chick Peas is another name for Garbanzo beans. They have been listed separate from other legumes because of their high nutritional value.

Garbanzo beans (like most legumes) have long been valued for their fiber content. Two cups provide the entire Daily Value! But the research news on garbanzos and fiber has recently taken us one step further by suggesting that the fiber benefits of garbanzo beans may go beyond the fiber benefits of other foods. In a recent study, two groups of participants received about 28 grams of fiber per day. But the two groups were very different in terms of their food sources for fiber. One group received dietary fiber primarily from garbanzo beans. The other group obtained dietary fiber from entirely different sources. The garbanzo bean group had better blood fat regulation, including lower levels of LDL-cholesterol, total cholesterol, and triglycerides.

In some parts of the world (for example, parts of India), garbanzo beans are eaten daily in large amounts and on a year-round basis. But a recent study has shown that we can obtain health benefits from garbanzo beans even when we eat much smaller amounts over a much shorter period of time. In this study, it took only one week of garbanzo bean consumption to improve participants' control of blood sugar and insulin secretion. Equally important, only one-third cup of the beans per day was needed to provide these blood-sugar related health benefits.

There's now direct evidence about garbanzo beans and appetite! Participants in a recent study reported more satisfaction with their diet when garbanzo beans were included, and they consumed fewer processed food snacks during test weeks in the study when garbanzo beans were consumed. They also consumed less food overall when the diet was supplemented with garbanzo beans.

PEANUTS

(*Arachis hypogaea*, Linn.)

Botanically these belong to the pulse tribe; leguminous seeds rich in nitrogenous matter, but for convenience, recipes for their use and cookery have been placed with nuts.

Peanuts are a mixed bag. Peanuts can be difficult to find in high-quality form; can be more commonly associated with adverse reactions than other foods; and can present more challenges to our food supply in terms of sustainability. Yet they can be very nutritious.

Peanuts are a very good source of monounsaturated fats, the type of fat that is emphasized in the heart-healthy Mediterranean diet. Studies of diets with a special emphasis on peanuts have shown that this little legume is a big ally for a healthy heart. In one such randomized, double-blind, cross-over study involving 22 subjects, a high monounsaturated diet that emphasized peanuts and peanut butter decreased cardiovascular disease risk by an estimated 21% compared to the average American diet.

In addition to their monounsaturated fat content, peanuts feature an array of other nutrients that, in numerous studies, have been shown to promote heart health. Peanuts are good sources of vitamin E, niacin, folate, protein and manganese. In addition, peanuts provide *resveratrol*, the phenolic antioxidant also found in red grapes and red wine that is thought to be responsible for the French paradox: the fact that in France, people consume a diet that is not low in fat, but have a lower risk of cardiovascular disease compared to the U.S. With all of the important nutrients provided by nuts like peanuts, it is no wonder that numerous research studies, including the Nurses' Health Study that involved over 86,000 women, have found that frequent nut consumption is related to reduced risk of cardiovascular disease.

A GROUP OF VEGETABLES CONTAINING NITROGENOUS MATTER WITHOUT STARCH OR SUGAR

Photos can be found at:

http://vegetables.healthyfoodseries.com/vegetables-containing-nitrogen-and-starch-2/

MUSHROOMS

All the mushrooms and truffles belong to a large group of fungi, plants void of chlorophyll. They are placed among the nitrogenous foods, that is they do not contain starch or sugar. They consist, however, of 90% water. Of the remaining 10% a portion is vegetable fibre. They are food adjuncts, or flavoring, rather than true foods.

They do not contain sufficient nitrogenous matter to take the place of meat. To obtain from them the proper amount of nourishment one would be obliged to eat them in large quantities; as they are dense and difficult of digestion, this would be impracticable and dangerous.

A cook-book is scarcely the proper place to discuss mushrooms; the subject is too large for the available space. A few recipes for the cooking and preserving of the more common varieties will, I am sure, be of great service.

The question, how can one be sure of "mushrooms" or "toadstools," is an important one. The average person calls

84

the edible varieties mushrooms, the poisonous ones toadstools.

The fact is, however, that they are all toadstools or all mushrooms. Some are poisonous, others edible. The question reverts then, to how can one be sure of knowing the poisonous from the edible varieties.

Let me emphatically state that there is no royal road to distinguishing the poisonous from the edible mushrooms; one must know all their characteristics, habitat and general appearance. All of the common tests, as the gold ring or silver spoon, are fallacies.

In certain parts of the country the common people use the *Morel*, calling it a mushroom and every other variety a toadstool. In many States the *Agaricus campestris* is known as the mushroom, and all others are toadstools. In Maine, especially on some of the coast islands, the *Cantharellus* is the mushroom. So that the term mushroom or toadstool is not applied to the same fungus in different places.

Avoid all mushrooms that have a veil hanging in a form of skirt from the stem and those having a cup or volva in the ground out of which the stem seems to be growing. While "veils" may be found on other mushrooms, they are sure to be 'found on the poisonous ones. Avoid such mushrooms; do not even taste them, for the poisonous ones are very deadly.

Mushrooms differ in analysis and density of flesh as well as in flavor, hence, different methods of cooking are desirable. The *Coprinus micaceus* and *Lepiota procera* are easily destroyed by long and severe cooking. The more dense and common *Agaricus campestris*, and some varieties of the

Boleti, require long slow cooking to make them tender, digestible, and bring out the flavor. Simplicity in seasoning is desirable; wine, mustard, onion or any other decided flavors will entirely overpower the delicate mushroom flavor.

All mushrooms are best cooked without peeling, with the exception of the puff ball, which should always be pared. In washing take one mushroom in each hand, gill sides down; wash them quickly by plunging them in and out of the water while rubbing the caps with the thumbs; shake and throw them into a colander.

Recipes for *Agaricus campestris* will answer for all other mushrooms which have firm, solid flesh, as the *Cantharellus, Agaricus Arvensis, Armillaria mellca, Paxillus rhodoxanthus, Hypholoma perplexum, Lactarius deliciosus, Lactarius volemus, Marasmius oreades*, and the *Russula. Russula virescens* is excellent raw, in salads. The *Coprini* are best baked or panned, the *Lepiota* broiled or panned, the *Morchella* (morel) stuffed and baked, the puff ball sliced and sautéd.

The *Agaricus campestris* grows in old pasture fields and along the roadside and often in gardens. It is usually found in the sod. The cap is first rounded, as it grows, expands and shows the gills, which are at first pink, growing a dark brown as the mushroom ages. The flesh is white, the gills are free from the stem, the flesh of both the cap and stem solid. It is the common pasture or meadow mushroom, and is, perhaps, the most widely known and collected of all mushrooms. It is this variety that is cultivated in cellars and caves.

COPRINUS, THE INKY MUSHROOM

Coprinus comatus is another well known variety of the more common mushrooms. These are found growing along railroads, especially where soft and hard coal are transported. Also in mining localities and on ash "dumps." In the soft coal districts of Illinois this mushroom grows most plentifully. It is readily recognized by its black spores. As it grows to maturity the gills seem to dissolve into a sort of inky fluid. The young plants or buttons have white gills which turn black as the spores mature. The cap has a rough shaggy appearance, hence, the common name, "shaggy mane." In appearance it is like a tiny umbrella closed down to the stem. The stem is hollow, loose from the cap and is easily taken out.

Coprinus atramentarius, the companion of the comatus, is also edible. The cap of this variety is smooth and does not so closely hug the stem. It also has white gills in a very young stage. The skin of the cap is smooth and of a grayish color, but in a short time it begins to spread and the gills turn very black from discoloration of the spores, and the edges begin to melt away. Both these varieties are not only edible, but exceedingly delicate and palatable. In the Eastern part of the United States they appear in the early summer, and continue until November. In Illinois they are most plentiful in September and October.

Coprinus micaceus, a tiny little mushroom, soft and easily digested, is another variety of this "inky" group. The caps of these are tan color, and the size of a large thimble.

They grow in huge groups around trees, especially elms. I have seen as many as two hundred in a single bunch. These are said to be the most easily digested of all mushrooms. They have black spores, as black as ink, after cooking.

LEPIOTA PROCERA

This is the "parasol" mushroom, or "Scotch bonnet." It grows in pastures, along the edges of woods, along roadsides at the edge of woods, and sometimes in the shady spots in gardens. The cap is oval at first, umbonate at the centre when expanded. When fully grown frequently measures from six to seven inches in diameter. The surface of the cap is reddish brown, in wet weather ofttimes quite pale. As the cap expands, the darker brown surface is torn and remains in scales all over the surface of the cap. The stem is round, "stuffed," and has a prominent ring just below the gills. This ring differs from a "veil" in that it is free from the stem and can be moved up and down. This variety is, of all mushrooms, the richest in flavor. They may be easily dried and are the best variety for catsup.

CLAVARIA

Clavaria or coral mushroom grows in large bunches in woods. One variety is saffron color, another white, another a bluish gray; all are exceedingly delicate and tender. These are best pickled or deviled.

CANTHARELLUS

This group is distinguished by the form of gills, which are decurrent, forked, sometimes irregular; in some species look like veins.

Cantharellus cibarius is known to most persons as the "chantarell," and is one of the best of the edible mushrooms. The entire mushroom, cap, gills and stem, is of a rich chrome yellow. When broken it has a faint odor of ripe peach. It grows in the woods, especially under hemlocks, generally in clusters of twos or threes. These are best stewed with cream.

MORCHELLA (Morels or Cup-Fungi)

These are different in shape from the ordinary mushrooms. The cap is cup shaped, the outside of which is covered with pits irregularly arranged. The Morchella esculenta is the one best known. It grows in orchards in the early spring.

These mushrooms may be stewed, baked or panned, but are best stuffed. Remove the stems, wash and drain. Make a stuffing of fine bread crumbs, seasoned with salt and pepper and chopped parsley and sufficient melted butter to moisten. Stuff the mushrooms; stand them in a baking pan, add a tablespoonful of butter and a half cup of stock. Bake thirty minutes, dish and put into the pan in which they were cooked one cupful of strained tomatoes. Boil rapidly fifteen minutes, or until slightly thickened, and strain it over the mushrooms. Garnish with triangular pieces of toast, and send at once to the table.

BEEFSTEAK (*Fistulina hepatica*)

This mushroom grows like a great red tongue on chestnut trees. It appears about August and continues until frost. The acid or sour taste makes them unpalatable alone, but as a sauce for beefsteak or for catsup they are excellent.

PUFF BALLS (*Lycoperdon*)

All puff balls are edible when young and fresh. The flesh must be white to the very centre. Do not use them if they have the slightest yellow tinge.

The giant puff ball (Lycoperdon giganteum) is the largest species of the genus. I have seen this variety in Indiana and Iowa weighing from seven to nine pounds.

BOLETUS

This group contains a large number of varieties. They belong to the same genera as the beefsteak mushrooms. The spores are not borne on gills as in the common mushrooms, but in pores or tubes; these pores give the under surface the appearance of a fine sponge. The flesh is soft and quickly decays.

To cook cut off the thick stem close to the pores. Wash the caps and remove the pores. Dust the caps with salt and pepper, dip them in beaten egg, roll in bread crumbs, and fry in hot fat. Serve at once with tomato catsup.

A GROUP OF VEGETABLES CONTAINING SUGAR, NO STARCH

Photos found at:
http://vegetables.healthyfoodseries.com/sugar-vegetables/

New, or green peas
Beets
New, or green corn
Carob beans

YOUNG GREEN PEAS

We don't usually think about green peas as an exotic food in terms of nutrient composition—but we should. Because of their sweet taste and starchy texture, we know that green peas must contain some sugar and starch (and they do). But they also contain a unique assortment of health-protective phytonutrients. One of these phytonutrients—a polyphenol called *coumestrol*--has recently come to the forefront of research with respect to stomach cancer protection.

Green peas stand out as an environmentally friendly food. Agricultural research has shown that pea crops can provide the soil with important benefits. First, peas belong to a category of crops called "nitrogen fixing" crops. With the help of bacteria in the soil, peas and other pulse crops are able to take nitrogen gas from the air and convert it into more complex and usable forms. This process increases nitrogen available in the soil without the need for added fertilizer. Peas also have a relatively shallow root system which can help prevent erosion of the soil, and once the peas have been picked, the plant remainders tend to break down relatively easily for soil replenishment. Finally, rotation of peas with other crops has been shown to lower the risk of pest problems. These environmentally friendly aspects of pea production add to their desirability as a regular part of our diet.

These are very rich in water, have little mineral matter, and if it were not for the sugar they contain would be placed with succulent vegetables. In menu building they are always served with starchy foods or meats. They are palatable and easy of digestion, when cooked simply. For invalids and children, however, they should be pressed through a colander to remove the hulls, and served either mashed or made into a purée.

COMPOSITION

Water 78.1
Proteid 4.0
Sugar 16.0
Fat 0.5
Cellulose 0.5
Mineral 0.9

Young peas are principally digested in the intestines.

BEETS
(*Beta vulgaris*, Linn.)

Both beets and Swiss chard are different varieties within the same plant family (*Amaranthaceae-Chenopodiaceae*) and their edible leaves share a resemblance in both taste and texture. Attached to the beet's green leaves is a round or oblong root, the part conjured up in most people's minds by the word "beet." Although typically a beautiful reddish-purple hue, beets also come in varieties that feature white, golden/yellow or even rainbow color roots. No matter what their color, however, beet roots aren't as hardy as they look; the smallest bruise or puncture will cause red beets' red-purple pigments (which contain a variety of phytonutrients including betalains and anthocyanins) to bleed, especially during cooking. Betalain pigments in beets are highly-water soluble, and they are also temperature sensitive. For both of these reasons, it is important to treat beets as a delicate food, even though they might seem "rock solid" and difficult to damage.

The ordinary beet root contains almost as much sugar as the white sugar beet that is grown for the purpose of making sugar. When young and tender, red beets are easily cooked, palatable and fairly digestible. For winter use it is far better to can young beets than to attempt to cook the old ones. They are dense and difficult of digestion even when cooked for hours. Beets are digested in the small intestines.

Beets are highly nutritious and "cardiovascular health" friendly root vegetables. Certain unique pigment antioxidants in the root as well as in its top greens have found to offer protection against coronary artery disease and stroke; lower cholesterol levels within the body, and have anti-aging effects.

The tops of young beets are boiled and served as greens. While they are without nourishment, they give variety to a spring diet, are palatable and good waste food.

Beets are a unique source of phytonutrients called betalains. Betanin and vulgaxanthin are the two best-studied betalains from beets, and both have been shown to provide antioxidant, anti-inflammatory, and detoxification support. The detox support provided by betalains includes support of some especially important Phase 2 detox steps involving glutathione. Although you can see these betalain pigments in other foods (like the stems of chard or rhubarb), the concentration of betalains in the peel and flesh of beets gives you an unexpectedly great opportunity for these health benefits.

COMPOSITION OF FULL
GROWN RED BEETS

```
Water . . . . . . . . . . . . . 82.2
Albuminoids . . . . . . . . . . . 0.4
Extractives, including amides . . . . 1.0
Sugar . . . . . . . . . . . . . 10.0
```

Pectose 2.4
Fat 0.1
Cellulose 3.0
Mineral matter 0.9

Health Benefits:

- Garden beet is very low in calories (provide only 45 kcal/100 g), and contain zero cholesterol and small amount of fat. Its nutrition benefits come particularly from fiber, vitamins, minerals, and unique plant derived anti-oxidants.
- The root is rich source of phytochemical compound, *glycine betaine.* These are very beneficial to the blood and vessels.
- Raw beets are an excellent source of folates. Folates are necessary for DNA synthesis within the cells. When given during peri-conception period folates can prevent neural tube defects in the baby.
- Fresh tubers contain small amounts of vitamin-C; however, its top greens are rather excellent sources of this vitamin. Vitamin C is one of the powerful natural antioxidants, which helps the human body scavenge deleterious free radicals one of the reasons for cancer development.
- Additionally, the top greens are an excellent source of carotenoids, flavonoid anti-oxidants, and vitamin A; contain these compounds several times more than that of in the roots. Vitamin A is required maintaining healthy mucus membranes

and skin and is essential for vision. Consumption of natural vegetables rich in flavonoids helps to protect from lung and oral cavity cancers.

- The root is also rich source of B-complex vitamins such as niacin (B-3), pantothenic acid (B-5), pyridoxine (B-6) and minerals such as iron, manganese, copper, and magnesium.
- Further, the root indeed has very good levels of potassium. Potassium lowers heart rate and regulates metabolism inside the cells by countering detrimental effects of sodium.

Selection and storage:

In the store, choose fresh, bright, firm textured beets with rich flavor and uniform size. Avoid those with slump looking or soft in consistency, over-mature and large. Whenever possible, go for organic to get maximum health benefits.

In the farmer markets, oftentimes the roots with intact top greens are for sale. If you are buying whole vegetable, cut the tops from its root as soon as possible since, they rob moisture and nutrition from the roots.

Beet greens, just like other greens, should be washed thoroughly in clean running water and rinsed in saline water for about 30 minutes in order to remove soil, sand, dirt, and any insecticide residues before use.

Top beet greens should be used while they are fresh. Beetroot, however, can be kept in the refrigerator set at high relative humidity for few weeks.

Preparation:

In addition to its crispy root, fresh tender top leaves and stems are also used for the preparation of recipes.

To prepare, gently scrub and wash the roots in clean running water before use in order to remove sand, soil, and dust. Peel the tough outer layer using a vegetable peeler. Cut the root into chunks, squares, or thin slices as you may desire.

Beet root may be eaten raw in salads. Steam small cubes and serve warm with butter. Pickled beets are a traditional food in the southern United States. Beet juice is a popular health drink. In India, the roots are eaten boiled in curries. In Europe, cooked chunks are eaten as a side dish with olive oil, vinegar or lemon juice. It is a popular in Eastern Europe as borscht (a soup).

YOUNG SWEET CORN

Sweet corn (*Zea mays convar. saccharata* var. *rugosa*; also called sugar corn and pole corn) is a variety of maize with a high sugar content. Sweet corn is the result of a naturally occurring recessive mutation in the genes which control conversion of sugar to starch inside the endosperm of the corn kernel. Unlike field corn varieties, which are harvested when the kernels are dry and mature (dent stage), sweet corn is picked when immature (milk stage) and prepared and eaten as a vegetable, rather than a grain. Since the process of maturation involves converting sugar to starch, sweet corn stores poorly and must be eaten fresh, canned, or frozen, before the kernels become tough and starchy.

Sugar or sweet corn is a variety of *Zea Mays*, used principally in America. It is palatable, contains but little nourishment, that mostly sugar, which is easily lost in the boiling. In fact, if the husks are removed, the sweetness is lost in a night, or if the ears are piled together one on top of the other for a few hours they heat, a slight fermentation takes place, changing the sugar, leaving the corn tasteless. It should be cooked immediately after picking, if possible.

To keep it overnight do not husk, but spread the ears out on a cool cellar floor or in the bottom of a cave or vault, or in the refrigerator.

Health Benefits:

- At 86 calories per 100 g, sugar corn kernels are moderately high in calories on comparison to other vegetables. However, fresh kernels have been much lower in calories than field corn and other cereals like wheat, rice, etc. Their calorie mainly comes from simpler carbohydrates like glucose, sucrose than complex sugars like amylose and amylopectin as in cereals.
- Sweet corn is gluten-free cereal and may be used safely much like rice, quinoa, etc., in celiac disease individuals.

- Corn features high-quality phyto-nutrition profile comprising of dietary fiber, vitamins, and antioxidants in addition to moderate proportions of minerals. It is one of the finest source dietary fibers. Together with slow digesting complex carbohydrates; moderate amounts of fiber in the food regulate a gradual rise in blood sugar levels. However, corn, in line with rice, potato, etc., is one of the high glycemic index food items, limiting its role as the chief food ingredient in diabetes patients.

- Yellow variety corn has significant levels of phenolic flavonoid pigment antioxidants such as *β-carotenes, and lutein, xanthins and cryptoxanthin* pigments along with vitamin A. Altogether; these compounds are required for maintaining healthy mucus membranes, skin and vision. Consumption of natural foods rich in flavonoids helps to protect from lung and oral cavity cancers.

- Corn is a good source of phenolic flavonoid antioxidant, ferulic acid. Several research studies suggest that ferulic acid plays vital role in preventing cancers, aging, and inflammation in humans.

- It also contains good levels of some of the valuable B-complex group of vitamins such as thiamin, niacin, pantothenic acid, folates, riboflavin, and pyridoxine. Many of these vitamins function as co-factors to enzymes during substrate metabolism.

- Further, it contains healthy amounts of some important minerals like zinc, magnesium, copper, iron, and manganese.

Selection and storage:

Sweet corn is a summer season crop in the temperate regions. However, it may be cultivated around the seasons in the tropical belt. In the US markets, fresh corn ears appear on the shelves by May and lasts until September. Fresh packs in the form of cobs or processed canned kernels may also be sold frozen in the markets all around the year. The cobs are generally available as yellow, white, or bicolor seed types. One may also collect them from neighborhood retailers or for even more enthusiasts may collect from the pick-your-own farms from the local farmers.

Fresh baby corns are usually come in small packages wrapped in plastic paper like button mushrooms. Choose to buy medium sized, firm, and fresh arrivals.

While buying, look for the well-formed ears with light green colored tight husks and clean, just about dry golden-brown silks. Gently pull down the husk from the tip-end to check for color as well as the milk-stage of kernels. You may buy fresh-husked cobs wrapped in plastic paper. Look for the harvest date; buy only if they are fresh as the kernels soon turn sugars to starch and lose their sweet, juicy flavor. Avoid if the husk is dry as it indicates the stock is old and hence out of flavor. Do not buy overtly matured cobs either.

Once at home, use them as early as possible. If you have to store, keep them inside the refrigerator, preferably along with its husk, to maintain flavor, taste, and moisture. They stay well for up to two to three days if stored at 90 percent humidity 32 °F.

Preparation:

To prepare, organic produce would not necessitate washing. Just remove the husk and silk and used as a vegetable. However, you may wash the de-husked cob in cold running water or dipping them in salt-water for about 15-20 minutes. Mop them dry using a paper towel.

Sweet-corn kernels can be used much like a vegetable rather than as a grain. In general, the whole cob may be served as a main dish. If you desired so to use only kernels in cooking, then using a paring knife slice through the kernels base all along the central woody-core to separate the them. Otherwise, you may remove individual kernels with the help your thumb as in the traditional way.

Farm fresh, raw sweet corn can be eaten as it is even without boiling or steaming.

The whole corncob may be grilled and served with salt and pepper seasoning.

The whole corncob may be steamed, or boiled in salt water and served with butter or oil.

Boiled kernels are an excellent accompaniment in salads, pizza, pasta, risotto, stews, omelets, fried-rice, etc.

Sweet corn soup and chowder are favorite starters in almost all corners of the world.

The water used for boiling the cob can be used along with onion, carrots, parsnip, celery-stalks, etc., in the preparation of delicious vegetable stock.

CAROB BEAN
(*Ceratonia siliqua*, Linn.)

The various names for Carob bean include locust bean, and St. John's bread—as it was likely the eaten by John the Baptist in the wilderness as in Biblical reference. Carob is used also for curing tobacco, in paper making, and as a stabilizer in food products. It has been claimed that the seeds were the original karat, the measurement of weight for precious jewels and metals. The pods filled with a sweet pulp, were eaten, fresh and dry and were a favorite food with the ancients. Specimens were exhumed Pompeii. The ancient Egyptians extracted a honey-like liquid from the hull of the pod in which they preserved fruits in Sicily, a spirit and a syrup are prepared.

Spanish missionaries introduced carob into Mexico and California. In 1854, seeds of this tree were distributed from the United States Patent Office and subsequently 8,000 seedlings were distributed around the US South. Many were later planted in Texas, Arizona, California and Florida as ornamental, shade trees.

High in carbohydrates, Carob has been used for its nutritional value for over centuries possibly millennia. Carob pods were the most important source of sugar before the spread of sugarcane and sugar beets.

Carob is naturally sweet and is similar to sweetened cocoa, but containing no caffeine, the obromine or other psychoactive substances. Unlike chocolate products, carob is non-toxic to dogs and is used in dog treats

Two distinct products are derived from its pod which is high in carbohydrate: carob bean gum and carob powder. Carob bean gum is made from the beans encased in the pod, used extensively in food manufacturing for binding. Carob powder, noted for its similarity to cocoa powder, is made by drying, roasting, and grinding the carob pod after the beans have been removed. The color and flavor of carob vary depending upon the roasting process—the longer carob is roasted, the darker its color and the blander its flavor. Solid carob, carob chips, and carob syrup are made from carob powder.

A GROUP OF GREEN OR SUCCULENT VEGETABLES

Photos found at:
http://vegetables.healthyfoodseries.com/green-or-succulent-vegetables/

A large group of vegetables, composed principally of water and mineral salts, of which the following are examples:

Artichokes
    Globe
    Jerusalem
    Cardoon
Asparagus
Bok Choy
Broccolli
Brussels sprouts
Cabbage
    White
    Red
Carrots
Cauliflower
Celeriac
Celery
Collards
Cucumbers
Dandelions
Dock shoots
Egg plant
Gherkin
Horseradish
Kale
Kohl-rabi

Leeks
Martynia
Moringa
Okra
Onions
Peppers
Radishes
Rhubarb
Ruta-baga
Savoy
Scallions
Spinach
Summer squash
Swiss chard
Tomatoes
Turnips
Vegetable marrow

The green or so-called succulent vegetables include many parts of plants, as shoots, leaves, stalks, stems and roots, and are valuable articles of food, not on account of the nutriment they contain, but for their succulent nature, the mineral salts they yield, and the flavor and variety they give to the daily bill of fare.

The true succulent vegetables, as a rule, do not contain nitrogenous matter of the sort that aids in the building of the tissues and flesh. Green vegetables are bulk foods, which aid in keeping up the natural peristaltic movement of the intestines. For this reason also they should be served at least once a day, each of the three hundred and sixty-five days of the year.

Many of these green vegetables contain materials physiologically suited to our needs; better by far take iron as we find it in many of the ordinary green vegetables, than from a bottle. Persons who cut from their diet all succulent vegetables are continuously taking pills to bring about the necessary natural conditions which would exist by the judicial and regular use of green vegetables.

The object of cooking non-starchy vegetables is to soften the fibre and to render them more easy of digestion. Green vegetables being very succulent easily part with their salts, and unless well cooked are unsightly as well as unpalatable, and common salt (chloride of sodium) does not in any way replace the mineral matter soaked and boiled from these vegetables. The common turnip, an admirable succulent vegetable, sightly, palatable and appetising if daintily cooked is, nine times out of ten, ruined in the cooking. Raw cabbage is digested in two hours and a half; after it passes through the hands of the ordinary cook it requires five hours, which certainly upsets the true definition of cooking. Besides making the cabbage difficult of digestion, careless cooking fills the house with an odor which is not only unpleasant but nauseating. The water is drained down the sink and a coarse unsightly dish without food value is the result. Vegetables with an odor, as cabbage and onions, should always be put over to cook in boiling salted water and cooked in an uncovered vessel.

Green vegetables lend themselves most easily to combinations of milk for the making of the so-called cream soups. The milk containing the needed nourishment is made palatable by the flavor of a few left-over vegetables. These soups are nitrogenous, easy of digestion and with whole wheat bread and butter form an admirable luncheon or supper dish for children. Save even a tablespoonful of vegetables that may be left from a meal; to-morrow add them to the soup; or mash and use them as flavoring to the meat or fish sauces. Among the best cream soups are potato, cream of corn, cream of pea, cream of beet and tomato. Spinach, kale or onions may be saved and added to cream sauces for fish and poultry.

TABLE OF ANALYSIS OF GREEN VEGETABLES IN COMMON USE

	Water	Albuminoids	Extractives	Gum	Fat	Celluose	Minner Matter	Sugar	Starch	Other Nitrogenous	
Artichokes Cardoon Globe Jerusalem	80.0	2.0		9.1	0.5	2.0	1.1	4.2			Inulin 1.1
Asparagus	89.8	3.0		1.8		2.6	0.9	1.5			Asparagin 0.4
Broccoli											
Brussels Sprouts	93.7	1.5			0.1		1.3				Carbohydrates 8.4
Cabbage	89.0	1.5		5.8	0.5	2.0	1.2				
Red	90.0	1.8			0.19	1.2	0.7				Ch. 5.8
Carrots	89.0	0.5		2.5	0.2	2.3	1.0	4.5			
Cauliflower	90.7	2.2		0.7		0.5	0.4	2.0			Ch. 4.7
Celeriac											
Celery	93.3	0.8				0.9	0.8	2.0		0.6	Mucilage & Starch 1.6
Collards											
Cucumbers	96.2	0.2		0.7		0.5	0.4	2.0			
Dandelion											
Dock											
Eggplant											
Horseradish											
Kale											
Kohi-rabi	87.1	2.6			0.2	1.3	1.5				Ch. 7.1
Leeks	91.8	1.2			0.5		0.7				Ch. 5.8
Okra											
Onions	91.0	1.5		4.8	0.2	2.0	0.5				
Peppers											
Radishes	90.8	1.4			0.1		0.7				Ch. 4.6
Ruta-baga											
Spinach	90.0	1.2			0.5	1.0	2.0				Ch. 4.0
Savoy	97.0	3.3			0.7	1.7	1.6				Ch. 6.0
Summer Squash											
Swiss											Ch. 8.9
Chard	82.9	3.8			0.9		3.5				
Tomatoes	89.8	1.4				1.3	0.8	6.0			Malic acid 0.7
Turnips	92.8	0.5	1.0	3.0	0.1	1.8	0.8				
Vegetable Marrow	94.8	0.6			0.2	1.3	0.5	2.0	0.6		

ARTICHOKES
GLOBE OR FRENCH

The artichoke (*Cynara Scolymus*, Linn.) a plant of the natural order of the *Composita*. The fleshy parts of the scales known as "choke," with prickly leaves around, constitute the portion used as food. In appearance these resemble the green cone of the pine tree, or a huge thistle.

This artichoke is a plant resembling a thistle, with a large scaly head like the cone of a pine. The receptacle underneath and the lower part of the leaves composing the head are the edible parts. It is an excellent and delicate vegetable.

Artichoke is one of the popular winter-season edible flower bud of the Mediterranean region known since ancient times for its medicinal and health benefiting qualities.

Globe artichoke grows up to 1.5-2 m tall, with arching, deeply lobed, silvery-green leaves about 0.5 m long. Beautiful light pink flowers develop in a large head from the edible buds. The bud is composed of compactly arranged triangular scales in a whorl fashion around a central "choke."

Artichoke globe measures about 6-10 cm in diameter and weighs about 150 g. Fuzzy; immature florets in the centre of the bud constitute its "choke." These are inedible in older, larger flowers. Edible portion of the buds consists primarily of the fleshy lower portions of the involucre bracts (triangular scales) and the base, known as the "heart."

Health Benefits:

- Artichoke is low in calories and fat; nonetheless, it is a rich source of dietary fiber. Dietary-fiber helps control constipation conditions, decrease bad or "LDL" cholesterol levels and helps prevent colon cancer risks.

- Artichoke contains bitter principles, *cynarin and sesquiterpene-lactones.* Scientific studies show that these compounds have overall cholesterol reduction in the blood.

- Fresh artichoke is an excellent source of vitamin *folic acid.* Scientific studies have proven that adequate levels of folates in the diet during pre-conception period, and during early pregnancy, help prevent neural tube defects in the newborn baby.

- Fresh globes also contain good amounts of anti-oxidant; *vitamin-C.* Regular consumption of foods rich in vitamin C helps the body develop resistance against infectious agents and scavenge harmful, pro-inflammatory free radicals from the body.

- It is one of the vegetable sources for *vitamin K.* Vitamin K has potential role bone health by promoting osteotrophic (bone formation) activity. Adequate vitamin-K levels in the diet help limiting neuronal damage in the brain; thus, has established role in the treatment of patients suffering from Alzheimer's disease.

- It is an also good source of antioxidants such as *silymarin, caffeic acid,* and *ferulic acid,* which help the body protect from harmful free-radical agents.

- It is also rich in B-complex group of vitamins such as niacin, vitamin B-6 (pyridoxine), thiamin, and pantothenic acid that are essential for optimum cellular metabolic functions.

- Further, artichoke is rich source of minerals like copper, calcium, potassium, iron, manganese and phosphorus. *Potassium* is an important component of cell and body fluids that helps controlling heart rate and blood pressure by countering effects of sodium. Manganese is used by the body as a co-factor for the antioxidant enzyme, *superoxide dismutase. Copper* is required in the production of red blood cells. *Iron* is required for red blood cell formation.

- Additionally, it contains small amounts of antioxidant flavonoid compounds like *carotene-beta, lutein, and zea-xanthin.*

Selection and storage:

Harvesting is usually done when the buds are still immature and picked just before the petals begin to open. Fresh globes are readily available in the market all around the season, although they are at their best during the springs.

112

In the store, choose fresh artichokes that feel heavy for their size and without any cuts or bruise. Its leaves should lie tight together, should feature dark green and squeak slightly when squeezed. Avoid very large, tough globes as they are unappetizing.

The globes best used while they are fresh. However, they can keep well if stored inside the refrigerator in a sealed plastic bag for up to a week.

Preparation:

Artichokes are a popular winter season vegetables throughout Europe. Small or baby artichokes can be eaten completely without removing the inside spiny choke.

To prepare bigger globes, rinse them in cold running water. Trim away the stem leaving about 1 inch from the base. Remove the lower layers of scales as they do not contain any flesh. Using a pair of scissors, trim the thorny scale ends. Trim the tip of the globe top using a paring knife up to an inch. Spread out the scales and then scrape off central choke. Rub a lemon slice over cut portion to prevent it from turning brown. Then, the globe is boiled in water upside down with some added salt and lemon juice until it gets soft.

To eat artichokes, take off individual leaf at a time, dip in your favorite sauce, and scrape off the fleshy base with your teeth. Center of leaf near its attachment to the heart holds more part that is edible.

Be sure to provide a plate to pile discarded leaves and finger bowl to wash hands for the guests!

JERUSALEM ARTICHOKES
(*Helianthus tuberosus*, Linn.)

These are the tubers of the so-called Italian sunflower, which grows wild and abundantly in many parts of the United States and Canada. They do not contain starch and but a trace of sugar; are fairly rich in carbohydrates of the gum series. They also contain inulin. Being free from starch they may be eaten uncooked; if properly cooked, however, they retain their crisp and tender conditions and are exceedingly palatable. They form one of the most important vegetables for diabetic patients.

ASPARAGUS
(*Asparagus officinalis*, Linn.)

The fleshy green spears of asparagus are both succulent and tender and have been considered a delicacy since ancient times. They were revered by ancient Greek and Romans. One of the oldest recorded vegetables; it is thought to have originated along the coastal regions of eastern Mediterranean and Asia Minor areas.

This highly prized vegetable arrives with the coming of spring, when its shoots break through the soil and reach their 6-8 inch harvest length

Asparagus belongs to the lily family. The plant is cultivated for the early shoots, which are in great favor both as a vegetable served hot, and cold as a salad.

Asparagus contains an alkaloid known as asparagin, and while it has a decided action upon the kidneys its true merits or demerits are not known.

Wild asparagus (*Asparagus racemosus*) is a species of asparagus with a long history of use in India and other parts of Asia as a botanical medicine. Many medicinal qualities of wild asparagus have been associated with phytonutrients present in its roots, and especially one type of phytonutrients called saponins. Recent research has shown that the species of asparagus most commonly consumed in the U.S. (*Asparagus officinalis*) also contains saponins, not only in its root portion put also in its shoots. Saponins found in common, everyday asparagus include asparanin A, sarsasapogenin, and protodioscin. Asparagus even contains small amounts of the diosgenin - one of the best-studied saponins that is especially concentrated in yam. Saponins in food have repeatedly been shown to have anti-inflammatory and anti-cancer properties, and their intake has also been associated with improved blood pressure, improved blood sugar regulation, and better control of blood fat levels.

Ingestion of young shoots may give an offensive smell to urine. This is due to the metabolism of *asparagusic acid*, which breaks down into various sulfur-containing degradation products. This odor last for a short time and is harmless.

Health Benefits:

- Asparagus is a very low calorie vegetable. 100 g fresh spears give only 20 calories.
- In addition, the spears contain moderate levels of dietary-fiber. Dietary fiber helps control constipation conditions, decrease bad (LDL) cholesterol levels and regulate blood sugar levels. Studies suggest that high-fiber diet help cut down colon-rectal cancer risks by preventing toxic compounds in the food from absorption.
- Its shoots have long been used in many traditional medicines to treat conditions like *dropsy* and *irritable bowel syndrome.*
- Fresh asparagus spears are the good source of anti-oxidants such as *lutein, zea-xanthin, carotenes*, and *crypto-xanthins*. This can help protect from possible cancer, neuro-degenerative diseases, and viral infections.
- Fresh asparagus are rich in folates. Scientific studies have shown that adequate consumption of folates in the diet during pre-conception period and during early pregnancy, help prevents neural tube defects in the newborn baby.
- The shoots are also rich in B-complex group of vitamins such as thiamin, riboflavin, niacin, vitamin B-6 (pyridoxine), and pantothenic acid

those are essential for optimum cellular enzymatic and metabolic functions.

- Fresh asparagus also contains fair amounts of anti-oxidant vitamins such as vitamin-C, vitamin-A, and vitamin-E. Regular consumption of foods rich in these vitamins helps the body develop resistance against infectious agents and scavenge harmful, pro-inflammatory free radicals from the body.

- Its shoots are also good source of vitamin K. Vitamin K has potential role bone health by promoting osteotrophic (bone formation) activity. Adequate vitamin-K levels in the diet help limiting neuronal damage in the brain; thus, has established role in the treatment of patients suffering from *Alzheimer's disease.*

- Asparagus is good in minerals, especially copper and iron. In addition, it has small amounts of some other essential minerals and electrolytes such as calcium, potassium, manganese, and phosphorus. *Potassium* is an important component of cell and body fluids that helps controlling heart rate and blood pressure by countering effects of sodium. Manganese is used by the body as a co-factor for the antioxidant enzyme, *superoxide dismutase. Copper* is required in the production of red blood cells. *Iron* is required for cellular respiration and red blood cell formation

Selection and storage:

Although one may find asparagus all around the season in the supermarkets, it is best available and is most flavorful in the springs. In Europe, its spears are sold in the shops from December until June.

Asparagus should be used as soon as possible after harvesting. Otherwise, it loses flavor since most of its sugar will be converted to starch. Therefore, purchase them from the local farms or farmer-markets whenever possible as they tend to be fresh and appetizing. In the markets select tender, firm, straight, smooth, uniform sized, dark green/purple stalks with tightly-closed tips. Avoid thick stalks with wide ridges in the stems, sunken or dull colored, as they indicate old stalk and hence, off flavored.

As its spears perish early, they should be harvested in the morning hours when air temperatures are cool. After picking, immerse them in ice-cold water to remove the heat; then drain the water and place the spears in plastic bags and store in the refrigerator at 38 to 40 degrees F with 90 to 95% relative humidity. At the higher temperatures, its spears lose natural sugar, vitamin-C, as well as flavor, and they become tough and begin to decay.

Preparation:

Fresh spears preferred in cooking. To prepare, wash them in cool running water with gentle scrub. Thin tender spears can be cooked directly. Thick stalks, however, may need peeling before used in the recipes.

In general, the spears need to be cooked briefly. In some households, traditional pots are used to cook asparagus where in its stalks immersed in boiling water while tips just allowed cooking by steam only.

Asparagus shoots are one of the most sought-after vegetables during the spring season.

Asparagus spears can be enjoyed raw, steamed, sautéed, stir-fried or mixed with vegetables, beans, poultry or seafood.

Steamed it can be served with melted butter, hollandaise sauce or parmesan cheese.

BOK CHOY

Bok choy or *leafy Chinese cabbage* is one of the popular mainland crops in China, Philippines, Vietnam and other oriental regions. Nonetheless, this humble Brassica family vegetable has gained popularity even in the western world for its sweet, succulent nutritious stalks.

In structure, bok choy resembles collards and could be described as a non-heading cabbage. It is basically a small plant which grows upright from the ground with smooth white romaine lettuce like stalks, which spread at the end to fine, glossy green, oval or round leaves. Full grown-up plant may reach about 12-18 inches in length.

Health Benefits:

- Bok choy is one of the popular leafy-vegetables very low in calories. Nonetheless, it is very rich source of many vital phyto-nutrients, vitamins, minerals and health-benefiting anti-oxidants.
- As in other Brassica family vegetables, bok choy too contains certain anti-oxidant plant chemicals like *thiocyanates, indole-3-carbinol, lutein, zea-xanthin, sulforaphane and isothiocyanates.* Along with dietary fiber, vitamins these compounds help to protect against breast, colon, and prostate cancers and help reduce LDL or "bad cholesterol" levels in the blood.
- Fresh bok chou is an excellent source of water-soluble antioxidant, vitamin-C. Regular consumption of foods rich in vitamin C helps the body develop resistance against infectious agents and scavenge harmful, pro-inflammatory free radicals.
- Bok-choy has more vitamin A, carotenes, and other flavonoid polyphenolic anti-oxidants than cabbage, cauliflower, etc.
- Bok-choy is a very good source of **vitamin K**, provides about 38% of RDA levels. Vitamin-K has a potential role in bone metabolism by promoting osteotrophic activity in bone cells. Further, vitamin-K also has established role in curing Alzheimer's disease patients by limiting neuronal damage in their brain.
- Fresh bok choy has many vital B-complex vitamins such as pyridoxine (vitamin B6), riboflavin,

pantothenic acid (vitamin B5), pyridoxine, and thiamin (vitamin B-1). These vitamins are essential in the sense that our body requires them from external sources to replenish.

- Further, this leafy vegetable is a moderate source of minerals, particularly calcium, phosphorous, potassium, manganese, iron and magnesium. Potassium is an important electrolyte in the cell and body fluids that helps regulate heart rate and blood pressure. Manganese is used by the body as a co-factor for the antioxidant enzyme, superoxide dismutase. Iron is required for the red blood cell formation.
- Like cabbage prolonged consumption of Bok choy can cause selling of the thyroid gland, known as goiter. It should therefore be used in moderation.

Selection and storage:

Although bok choy is available year-round, it is best during winter season. In the markets, buy fresh harvest featuring firm stalks and dark green crispy flavorful leaves. Avoid slump plant with leaves wilted and lost their luster.

Once at home store whole bok-choy in the vegetable compartment in the refrigerator set at high relative humidity. If stored appropriately, it stays fresh for up to 3-4 days without the loss of much of nutrients. However, bok-choy is more nutritious, sweeter, and flavorful when used fresh.

Preparation:

Trim the base and remove outer discolored leaves. Wash the whole vegetable in cold water. Gently pat dry or place it upside down until all the water drained out.

To prepare, separate outer stalks from the base using a paring knife and slice the whole plant in equal halves lengthwise. Then, chop from the stem end about an inch apart and work towards its leafy end. Add it in to a variety of recipes either combined with other vegetables or enjoy all alone in stir-fry or soup.

Bok choy stalks can be eaten raw, added to salads or sandwiches.

Baby bok choy can be a very attractive addition to salads and stir-fries.

In Eastern Asia, it is used much like cabbage in stew fries.

It is used in many modern-day recipes like stir fries, soups, etc.

BROCCOLI

Broccoli is a member of the cabbage family, and is closely related to cauliflower. Its cultivation originated in Italy. *Broccolo*, its Italian name, means "cabbage sprout." Broccoli's name is derived from the Latin word brachium, which means branch or arm, a reflection of its tree-like shape that features a compact head of florets attached by small stems to a larger stalk. Because of its different components, this vegetable provides a complex of tastes and textures, ranging from soft and flowery (the florets) to fibrous and crunchy (the stem and stalk). Its color can range from deep sage to dark green to purplish-green, depending upon the variety. One of the most popular types of broccoli sold in North America is known as Italian green, or Calabrese, named after the Italian province of Calabria where it first grew.

It's no coincidence that more than 300 research studies on broccoli have converged in one unique area of health science—the development of cancer—and its relationship to three metabolic problems in the body. Those three problems are (1) chronic inflammation (2) oxidative stress, and (3) inadequate detoxification. While these types of problems have yet to become part of the public health spotlight, they are essential to understanding broccoli's unique health benefits. Over the past 5 years, research has made it clear that our risk of cancer in several different organ systems is related to the combination of these three problems.

Broccoli is a cool-season crop and demands fertile rich and well-drained soil to flourish. Technically; broccoli is categorized into two main types according to their appearance; heading and sprouting. Heading variety forms a large, solid head, whereas sprouting types forms many smaller heads or florets.

Mature plant bears about 4-10 inches wide, dark green to purple color flower-head depending on the cultivar type. Its central thick stalk measures about 6-10 inches in length. Both stalk and fleshy flower heads are edible.

Health Benefits:

- Broccoli is one of the very low calorie vegetables; provide just 34 calories per 100 g. Nevertheless, it is rich in dietary fiber, minerals, vitamins, and anti-oxidants that have proven health benefits.
- Fresh Broccoli is a storehouse of many phytonutrients such as *thiocyanates, indoles, sulforaphane, isothiocyanates* and *flavonoids like beta-carotene cryptoxanthin, lutein, and zea-xanthin*. Studies have shown that these compounds help protect from prostate, colon, urinary bladder, pancreatic, and breast cancers.
- Fresh vegetable is exceptionally rich source of vitamin-C. Vitamin-C is a powerful natural anti-oxidant and immune modulator, helps fight against flu causing viruses.
- Further, it contains very good amounts of another anti-oxidant vitamin, vitamin-A. Together with other pro-vitamins like beta-carotene, alpha-carotene, and zea-xanthin, vitamin A helps maintain integrity of skin and mucus membranes. Vitamin A is essential for healthy eye-sight and helps prevent from macular degeneration of the retina in the elderly population.
- Broccoli leaves (green tops) are an excellent source of carotenoids and vitamin A.
- Fresh broccoli heads are an excellent source of folates. Studies have shown that consumption of fresh

vegetables and fruits rich in folates during pre-conception, and pregnancy helps prevent neural tube defects in the offspring.

- This flower vegetable is rich source of vitamin-K; and B-complex group of vitamins like niacin (vit B-3), pantothenic acid (vit.B-5), pyridoxine (vit.B-6), and riboflavin. The flower heads also have some amount of omega-3 fatty acids.
- It is also a good source of minerals like calcium, manganese, iron, magnesium, selenium, zinc and phosphorus.
- Broccoli is like cabbage and may cause swelling of the thyroid gland in some individuals. However most people should be able to eat regularly.

Selection and storage:

Fresh broccoli heads are available year around. In the store, choose fresh, bright, compact, firm textured flower heads with rich flavor. Avoid those with over matured featuring yellow flower buds, excessive branches and hollow stem. Whenever possible, go for organic farm products to get maximum health benefits.

Once at home, rinse flower heads by dipping it upside down in salt water for up to 30 minutes and then clean in running cold water before use in order to remove any pesticide residues and dust. Broccoli greens should also be treated in the same way as you do in washing any other greens like spinach.

Whenever possible, eat broccoli while they are fresh. Otherwise, it can be placed in the refrigerator wrapped in a zip pouch where it may keep well for a few days.

Preparation:

Fleshy flower heads, stalks and leaves are edible. Broccoli sections are being used in varieties of delicacies. Tough stalks and thick leaves are trimmed using paring knife.

Young, tender, broccoli heads may be eaten raw or as salad.

The flower heads are great in stir fries and can also be steamed.

Microwaving can destroy some heat sensitive vitamins.

BRUSSELS SPROUTS

Brussels sprouts are members of the Brassica family and therefore kin to broccoli and cabbage. They resemble miniature cabbages, with diameters of about 1 inch. They grow in bunches of 20 to 40 on the stem of a plant that grows as high as three feet tall. Brussels sprouts are typically sage green in color, although some varieties feature a red hue. They are oftentimes sold separately but can sometimes be found in stores still attached to the stem. Perfectly cooked Brussels sprouts have a crisp, dense texture and a slightly sweet, bright, and "green" taste.

Brussels sprouts are winter crops and flourish well in cool weather.

Health Benefits:

- The sprouts are one of the low-glycemic nutritious vegetables that should be considered in weight reduction programs.
- Brussels sprouts are a storehouse of several flavonoid anti-oxidants like *thiocyanates, indoles, lutein, zea-xanthin, sulforaphane* and *isothiocyanates.* Together, these phytochemicals offer protection from prostate, colon, and endometrial cancers.
- Di-indolyl-methane (DIM), a metabolite of *indole-3-carbinol* is found to be an effective immune modulator, anti-bacterial and anti-viral agent through its action of potentiating "Interferon-γ" receptors.
- In addition, brussel sprouts contain glucoside, sinigrin. Early laboratory studies suggest that *sinigrin* help protect from colon cancers by destroying pre-cancerous cells.
- Brussel sprouts are an excellent source of **vitamin C.** Together with other antioxidant vitamins such as vitamin A and E, it helps protect the body by trapping harmful free radicals.
- Zea-xanthin, an important dietary carotenoid in sprouts, is selectively absorbed into the retinal macula-lutea in the eyes where it is thought to provide anti-oxidant and protective light-filtering functions from UV rays. Thus, it helps prevent retinal damage,

"age-related macular degeneration related macular degeneration disease" (ARMD), in the elderly.

- Sprouts are the good source of another anti-oxidant vitamin A. Vitamin A is required for maintaining healthy mucus membranes and skin and is essential for acuity of vision. Foods rich in this vitamin have been found to offer protection against lung and oral cavity cancers.

- It is one of the excellent vegetable sources for vitamin-K. Vitamin K has potential role bone health by promoting osteotrophic (bone formation and strengthening) activity. Adequate vitamin-K levels in the diet help limiting neuronal damage in the brain and thereby, preventing or at least, delay the onset of Alzheimer's disease.

- Further, the sprouts are notably good in many B-complex groups of vitamins such as niacin, vitamin B-6 (pyridoxine), thiamin, pantothenic acid, etc., that are essential for substrate metabolism inside the human body.

- They are also rich source of minerals like copper, calcium, potassium, iron, manganese, and phosphorus. 100 g fresh sprouts provide 25 mg (1.5% of RDA) sodium and 389 mg (8% of RDA) potassium. Potassium is an important component of cell and body fluids that helps controlling heart rate and blood pressure by countering effects of sodium. Manganese is used by the body as a co-factor for the antioxidant enzyme, *superoxide dismutase*. Iron is required for cellular oxidation and red blood cell formation.

- Being Brassica family, they may cause swelling of thyroid gland and should be avoided by those with thyroid dysfunction. Healthy individuals may be able to consume liberally.

Selection and storage:

Brussel sprouts are cool season vegetables. In general, sprouts are harvested when the lower buds mature and reach about an inch in size. Fresh sprouts should feature firm, compact and dark green. Avoid sprouts featuring loose leaf, yellowish and light in hand.

Fresh sprouts keep well in the refrigerator for up to a day or two. Remove any damaged or discolored outer leaves and store fresh unwashed sprouts in plastic bags/zip pouches in the vegetable container in the refrigerator.

Preparation:

Before cooking, remove discolored and loosen outer leaves and the stems are trimmed. Wash in clean water and then, soak for few minutes in salt water to remove any dust particles and insect's eggs.

Fresh sprouts are delicate in flavor, however, overcooking results in the release of *allyl isothiocyanates* imparting sulfurous odor (pungent smell) to cooked recipes. Therefore, sprouts are generally blanched in boiling water for just about 5 minutes, cooled and then added to the recipes.

Sprouts can be cooked by boiling, microwaving or steaming.

Roasted and salted sprouts are a favorite snack in Europe.

CABBAGE

Under this heading will be considered all the varieties of the single species (*Brassica oleracea*, Linn.) a most variable plant belonging to the Mustard Family. By selection and cultivation the whole cabbage tribe has been evolved from one plant. All of these plants contain a volatile oil, rich in hydrogen and sulphur, which is driven off by careless cooking. The odor is unpleasant and particularly penetrating; in fact, badly cooked cabbage may be traced by this odor to the house a square away. Such cabbage is not only difficult of digestion but has lost its color and flavor, and is really unfit for food. Carefully boiled cabbage is delicate, quite easy of digestion, and is white and sightly.

Plants belonging to this family, like all green vegetables, should be cooked in salted boiling water in an uncovered vessel.

Researchers now realize that different types of cabbage (red, green, and Savoy) contain different patterns of glucosinolates. This new knowledge means that your broadest health benefits from cabbage are likely to come from inclusion of all varieties in your diet.

In one recent study, short-cooked and raw cabbage were the only types of cabbage to show cancer-preventive benefits—long-cooked cabbage failed to demonstrate measurable benefits.

HEAD CABBAGE

In this plant the leaves have by cultivation been crowded into a large dense head.

Cabbage is a waste food, principally digested in the intestines, more easily digested raw than boiled; if carefully cooked in salted water it is, however, quite as readily digested as when raw. Finely shredded, with French dressing, it makes an admirable dinner salad. The head of a "winter" cabbage being very dense, excludes the sun and the cabbage is said to be bleached and tender.

RED CABBAGE

Red cabbage forms into hard heads the same as white cabbage; it is not, however, so delicate or valuable, as the coloring matter fades in the cooking. It is used principally for pickling, although the Germans make it into one or two very palatable dishes.

Health Benefits:

- Fresh, dark green-leafy cabbage is incredibly nutritious; however, very low in fat and calories.

- The vegetable is the storehouse of phyto-chemicals like *thiocyanates, indole-3-carbinol, lutein, zea-xanthin, sulforaphane, and isothiocyanates.* These compounds are powerful antioxidants and known to help protect against breast, colon, and prostate cancers and help reduce LDL or "bad cholesterol" levels in the blood.

- Fresh cabbage is an excellent source of natural antioxidant, vitamin C. Regular consumption of foods rich in vitamin C helps the body develop resistance against infectious agents and scavenge harmful, pro-inflammatory free radicals.

- It is also rich in essential vitamins such as pantothenic acid (vitamin B-5), pyridoxine (vitamin B-6) and thiamin (vitamin B-1). These vitamins are essential in the sense that our body requires them from external sources to replenish.

- It also contains an adequate amount of minerals like potassium, manganese, iron, and magnesium. Potassium is an important component of cell and body fluids that helps controlling heart rate and blood pressure. Manganese is used by the body as a co-factor for the antioxidant enzyme, *superoxide dismutase.* Iron is required for the red blood cell formation.

- Cabbage is a very good source of vitamin K. Vitamin-K has the potential role in bone metabolism by promoting osteotrophic activity in them. So enough vitamin K in the diet gives you healthy bones. In addition, vitamin-K also has established role in curing Alzheimer's disease patients by limiting neuronal damage in their brain.

Selection and storage:

Cabbage is a cool-season crop. In the US supermarkets, however one may find them a year around. While buying, choose fresh, compact, firm, medium-size head heavy for its size.

Pests are common in cabbage. Conventionally grown heads may be subjected to insecticide spray to avoid pest infestation. Therefore, wash thoroughly in running water then soak in saline water for about 30 minutes, again wash in clean water in order to remove dust, pests, eggs/ova/cysts and any residual insecticides.

Use cabbage while farm fresh to get its maximum health benefits. However, it can be stored in the refrigerator for few days for later use.

Preparation:

To prepare, trim off the stem end and discard any withered outer layer leaves. Wash the head as described above. Cut the head into two equal halves and then slice the leaves as you may desire in the recipes.

Cleaned cabbage can be eaten raw.

Sliced or grated raw leaves can be added to salad.

Fresh or pickled cabbage leaves used as rolls are popular in Central Europe, Balkans and Asia minor.

Stew fried cabbage is favorite dishes in China and South East Asia.

CARROTS
(*Daucus Carota*, Linn.)

Carrots belong to the *Umbelliferae* family, named after the umbrella-like flower clusters that plants in this family produce. As such, carrots are related to parsnips, fennel, parsley, anise, caraway, cumin and dill. Carrots can be as small as two inches or as long as three feet, ranging in diameter from one-half of an inch to over two inches. Carrot roots have a crunchy texture and a sweet and minty aromatic taste, while the greens are fresh tasting and slightly bitter. While we usually associate carrots with the color orange, carrots can actually be found in a host of other colors including white, yellow, red, or purple. In fact, purple, yellow and red carrots were the only color varieties of carrots to be cultivated before the 15th or 16th century.

As a result of cultivation this root has grown fleshy, succulent, and of a light yellow or pale orange color. When young and fresh it is sweet, tender and agreeable; but becomes hard and strong when old. Carrots cut into thin slices and roasted are used as a coffee substitute or "'extract" in this country and in many parts of Germany. When roasted and boiled with water they yield a yellow liquid used as butter coloring. Full grown or mature carrots are quite rich in sugar and contain some starch. The young succulent roots, however, contain but little more than water and mineral matter. They have a trace of iron and are said to be anti-scorbutic.

Carrots are perhaps best known for their rich supply of the antioxidant nutrient that was actually named for them: beta-carotene. However, these delicious root vegetables are the source not only of beta-carotene, but also of a wide variety of antioxidants and other health-supporting nutrients. The areas of antioxidant benefits, cardiovascular benefits, and anti-cancer benefits are the best-researched areas of health research with respect to dietary intake of carrots.

Health Benefits:
- Sweet and succulent carrots are notably rich in anti-oxidants, vitamins and dietary fiber; however, they provide only 41 calories per 100 g, negligible amount of fat and no cholesterol.
- They are exceptionally rich source of carotenes and vitamin-A. Studies have found that flavonoid compounds in carrots help protect from skin, lung and oral cavity cancers.
- Carrots are rich in poly-acetylene antioxidant falcarinol. has found that *falcarinol* in carrots may help fight against cancers by destroying pre-cancerous cells in the tumors.

135

- Fresh roots are also good in vitamin C. Vitamin C helps the body maintain healthy connective tissue, teeth and gum. Its anti-oxidant property helps the body protect from diseases and cancers by scavenging harmful free radicals.
- Carrots are rich in many B-complex groups of vitamins such as folic acid, vitamin B-6 (pyridoxine), thiamin, pantothenic acid, etc., that acts as co-factors to enzymes during substrate metabolism in the body.
- They also compose healthy levels of minerals like copper, calcium, potassium, manganese and phosphorus. Potassium is an important component of cell and body fluids that helps controlling heart rate and blood pressure by countering effects of sodium. Manganese is used by the body as a co-factor for the antioxidant enzyme, *superoxide dismutase.*

Selection and storage:

Although carrots are available throughout the year, locally grown carrots are in season in the summer and fall when they are the freshest and most flavorful. When buying, look for young, tender, bright-colored roots with firm consistency. Avoid soft, flabby roots, with cuts or mold. Furthermore, avoid very large-sized roots as they indicate over maturity; resulting in their poor eating quality.

Excessive sun light exposure of the root above ground can result in greenish discoloration near the top end due to chlorophyll photo-pigment deposition. Although this may not affect health badly, however, it depletes sweet taste of the roots. Forking or twisted carrots may be the indication of either disease infestation or close crop cultivation.

Once at home, wash them thoroughly in water to remove dust, soil, or insecticide/fungicides. Generally, the top greens are trimmed from the root and stored in the vegetable compartment of the refrigerator where they keep well for 1-2 weeks. Set refrigerator temperature level below 35 degree F and high humidity to maintain vitality.

Preparation:

Wash carrots thoroughly before use. Trim both ends; gently scrape off outer skin and smaller hairy roots. The younger roots have crispy, pleasant taste, and rich flavor. Raw carrots are naturally sweet and juicy; however, boiling them in water for few minutes enriches their flavor and enhances the bioavailability of nutrients.

Fresh carrots can be enjoyed as is or can be used raw in salads.

Carrot juice is delicious and can be used alone or with fruit juice.

Carrots blend well with vegetables like green beans, potato, peas in stews, stir fries, etc.

The carrot root can be used in preparation of cakes, tarts, puddings, soups, etc.

Carrots are also used in the preparation of healthy baby foods.

CAULIFLOWER

Cauliflower, a cruciferous vegetable, is in the same plant family as broccoli, kale, cabbage and collards. It has a compact head (called a "curd"), with an average size of six inches in diameter, composed of undeveloped flower buds. The flowers are attached to a central stalk. When broken apart into separate buds, cauliflower looks like a little tree, something that many kids are fascinated by.

Cauliflower and broccoli have all the nutritious matter concentrated in a short, compact bunch of flowers formed into a soft head. Broccoli is both white and purple, but the name is usually applied to the loose heads of cauliflower. Broccoli is more hardy than cauliflower and is said to be rather more easily digested. Both may be prepared and served according to the same rules. Broccoli with chicken stock is frequently made into mock bisque soup. The brilliant pink makes it a desirable soup for pink luncheons or dinners. Both cauliflower and broccoli are more delicate and easily digested than common cabbage.

While cauliflower is not a well-studied cruciferous vegetable from a health standpoint, you will find several dozen studies linking cauliflower-containing diets to cancer prevention, particularly with respect to the following types of cancer: bladder cancer, breast cancer, colon cancer, prostate cancer, and ovarian cancer. This connection between cauliflower and cancer prevention should not be surprising, since cauliflower provides special nutrient support for three body systems that are closely connected with cancer development as well as cancer prevention. These three systems are (1) the body's detox system, (2) its antioxidant system, and (3) its inflammatory/anti-inflammatory system. Chronic imbalances in any of these three systems can increase risk of cancer, and when imbalances in all three systems occur simultaneously, the risk of cancer increases significantly.

Health Benefits:

- It is very low in calories. 100 g of the fresh cauliflower head provides only 26 calories. Nevertheless, it comprises of several health-benefiting antioxidants and vitamins in addition to be very low in fat and contains no cholesterol.

- Its florets contain about 2 g of dietary fiber per 100 g.

- Cauliflower contains several anti-cancer phyto-chemicals like *sulforaphane* and plant sterols such as *indole-3-carbinol,* which appears to function as an anti-estrogen agent. Together these compounds have proven benefits against prostate, breast, cervical, colon, ovarian cancers by virtue of their cancer-cell growth inhibition, cytotoxic effects on cancer cells.

- Furthermore, *Di-indolyl-methane (DIM),* which has found effective as immune modulator, anti-bacterial and anti-viral compound by synthesis and potentiating Interferon-Gamma receptors. DIM has currently been found application in the treatment of recurring respiratory papillomatosis caused by the Human Papilloma Virus (HPV) and is in Phase III clinical trials for cervical dysplasia.

- Fresh cauliflower is an excellent source of vitamin C. Vitamin-C is a proven antioxidant helps fight against harmful free radicals, boosts immunity and prevents from infections and cancers.

- It contains good amounts of many vital B-complex groups of vitamins such as folates, pantothenic acid (vitamin B5), pyridoxine (vitamin B6) and thiamin (vitamin B1), niacin (B3) as well as vitamin K. These vitamins are essential in the sense that body requires them from external sources to replenish and required for fat, protein and carbohydrate metabolism.

- It is an also good source of minerals such as manganese, copper, iron, calcium and potassium. Manganese is used in the body as a co-factor for the antioxidant enzyme, *superoxide dismutase*. *Potassium* is an important intracellular electrolyte helps counter the hypertension effects of sodium.

Selection and storage:

Cauliflowers are available all year around; however, they are at their best during winter months. In general, harvesting done when the head reaches the desired size but before the buds begin to separate.

In the stores, choose fresh heads featuring snow/creamy white, compact, even heads that feel heavy in hand. Grainy surface and separate heads indicate over maturity while green coloration may be due to over exposure to sunlight. Avoid heads with bruised surface as they indicate poor handling of the flower and those with dark color patches as they indicate mold disease known as downy mildew.

Once at home, store in the refrigerator set with higher relative humidity. They stay fresh for about a week if stored properly.

Preparation:

Its creamy-white flower heads are favored in variety of delicacies world-wide. To wash, place head upside down rinsed in a large bowl of cold water or salt water brine for about 15-20 minutes to ensure removal of any insects, soil or fungicide/insecticide sprays. Gently pat dry using soft cloth. Remove tough stem and leaves.

Usually florets cut into equal sections to help cook evenly. Cook covered in a little boiled salted water until tender for few minutes. Overcooking may result in loss of nutrients, especially vitamin-C.

Cauliflower mixes well with vegetables, lentils and meat.

Its florets can be added in pasta bake, casseroles and to make curry/soup.

It is also widely used in pickling.

CELERIAC
(*Apium graveolens*, Variety *Rapaceum*)

Celeriac, or turnip rooted celery, is a variety of the common white celery of which the root is enlarged and edible — not the stalks, as in the common celery. These roots are peeled, sliced, boiled and served cold with mayonnaise dressing under the name of celery root salad.

CARDOON
(*Cynara Carduncuhis*, Linn.)

This plant resembles the artichoke; the edible portion, however, consists of the thick, fleshy leaf stalks and midribs bleached. The bleaching is done by tying up the leaves, wrapping all but the top to exclude the sun.

These are boiled in salted water and served the same as asparagus, with cream sauce or sauce Hollandaise.

The term **"Chard"** is applied to the leaf stalks and midrib of the globe artichoke, which are tied and bleached in the same manner as cardoons. These are also boiled and served with sauce Hollandaise.

CELERY
(*Apium graveolens*, Linn.)

In most U.S. markets, it's the Pascal family of greenish to pale-green celery cultivars that we've become most accustomed to finding in the produce section. Pascal celery is larger than most other celery types, with firm, solid stalks and leafy ends. Yet even within this particular scientific type of celery (*Apium graveolens* var. *dulce*), there are many other options including Matador, Red Stalk, Tango, and Sonora. Celery actually comes in a variety of colors from sheer white to vibrant gold to rich red and deep green.

Regardless of which celery variety you choose to buy or grow, there are nutrient benefits to be found in all parts of the plant, including the leaves, stalks, roots, and seeds. "Celery hearts" usually refers to the innermost stalks of Pascal celery. These stalks are typically the most tender.

Celery has by cultivation lost its acrid taste, and become sweet and mild. To make it still more agreeable, the gardener banks the earth around the stalks as they grow until all but the tops are covered; in this way the sun is excluded and the stems are bleached, succulent and tender. As soon as celery comes home from the market or is brought into the house, cut off the green tops and put them aside for soup flavoring; separate the heads, saving the outside green pieces for stewing or celery sauce, and the very tender inner portion for eating raw.

Celery will keep much longer if the stalks are placed in a deep jar of cold water. The very large varieties are best for stewing; for eating raw, the small inferior looking heads are usually the sweetest.

Celery is an important food source of conventional antioxidant nutrients, including vitamin C, beta-carotene, and manganese. But its "claim to fame" in terms of antioxidant nutrients may very well be its phytonutrients. Many of these phytonutrients fall into the category of phenolic antioxidants and have been shown to provide anti-inflammatory benefits as well. Below is a representative list of the phenolic antioxidants found in celery.

COLLARDS

Collards are leafy green vegetables that belong to the same family that includes cabbage, kale, and broccoli. While they share the same botanical name as kale, Brassica oleracea, and some resemblance, they have their own distinctive qualities. Like kale, collards are one of the non-head forming members of the Brassica family. Collards' unique appearance features dark blue green leaves that are smooth in texture and relatively broad. They lack the frilled edges that are so distinctive to their cousin kale.

Long a staple of the Southern United States, collard greens, unlike their cousins kale and mustard greens, have a very mild, almost smoky flavor. Although they are available year-round they are at their best from January through April.

The cholesterol-lowering ability of collard greens may be the greatest of all commonly eaten cruciferous vegetables. In a recent study, steamed collard greens outshined steamed kale, mustard greens, broccoli, Brussels sprouts, and cabbage in terms of its ability to bind bile acids in the digestive tract. When this bile acid binding takes place, it is easier for the bile acids to be excreted from the body. Since bile acids are made from cholesterol, the net impact of this bile acid binding is a lowering of the body's cholesterol level. It's worth noting that steamed collards show much greater bile acid binding ability than raw collards.

144

Several cultivar types of collard greens are grown around the planet depending on the soil type, climate, etc.

1. Blue Max: It has very attractive savoy- like blue-green leaves.
2. Georgia: It is also known as Georgia LS or Georgia Southern. It has blue-green and slightly savoy-leaves.
3. Vates: Plant is compact and leaves are smooth and dark green.
4. Champion: Low growing plant, featuring smooth, dark-green leaves with short internodes.
5. Flash: It is a very uniform Vates type with smooth, dark-green leaves.
6. Heavy-Crop: It has very large, slightly savoy like, blue-green leaves. Leaves have close internodes spacing so bunching can be more difficult.

Health Benefits:

- Collard leaves are very low in calories (provide only 30 calories per 100 g) and contain no cholesterol. However, its green leaves contain a very good amount of soluble and insoluble dietary fiber that offer protection against hemorrhoids, constipation as well as colon cancer diseases.
- Widely considered to be wholesome foods, collards are rich in invaluable sources of phyto-nutrients with potent anti-cancer properties, such as di-indolyl-methane (DIM) and *sulforaphane* that have proven benefits against *prostate, breast,*

cervical, colon, ovarian cancers by virtue of their cancer-cell growth inhibition and cytotoxic effects on cancer cells.

- *Di-indolyl-methane* has also found to be effective immune modulator, anti-bacterial and anti-viral properties by potentiating Interferon-gamma receptors.

- The leaves are also an excellent source of folates. Folates are important in DNA synthesis and when given during the peri-conception period can prevent neural tube defects in the baby.

- Fresh collard leaves are also rich in vitamin-C. Vitamin-C is a powerful natural anti-oxidant that offers protection against free radical injury and flu-like viral infections.

- Collard greens are an excellent source of vitamin-A and carotenoid anti-oxidants such as *lutein, carotenes, zea-xanthin, crypto-xanthin,* etc. These compounds are scientifically found to have antioxidant properties. Vitamin A also required maintaining healthy mucus membranes and skin and is also essential for healthy vision. Consumption of natural fruits rich in flavonoids helps to protect from lung and oral cavity cancers.

- This leafy vegetable contains amazingly high levels of vitamin-K. Vitamin K has a potential role in the increase of bone mass by promoting osteotrophic activity in the bone. It also has the beneficial effect in Alzheimer's disease patients by limiting neuronal damage in their brain.

- Collards are rich in many vital B-complex groups of minerals such as niacin (vitamin B-3), pantothenic acid (vitamin B-5), pyridoxine (vitamin B-6) and riboflavin.
- Further, the leaves and stems are good in minerals like iron, calcium, copper, manganese, selenium and zinc.
- Collards like other members of the Brassica family can cause swelling of the thyroid gland. This should only affect those with thyroid conditions.

Selection and storage:

Although fresh collard greens are available year around in the stores, they are at their best from November through April. The plant is generally ready to harvest at 6-8 weeks after planting. Generally the whole plant is cut about 4 inches from the ground and sent to market in bunches. Usually, the cut ends sprouts again and bears new stems from the sides which can then be harvested again after few weeks.

In the stores, look for fresh, bright, crispy leaves with stout stalk. Avoid those with yellow discolored, sunken leaves. Whenever possible, choose these greens from the nearby organic farm in order to get maximum health benefits.

Once at home, collard greens should be cleaned as the same way as you do in any other greens like spinach. Wash the whole bunch in cold running water for few minutes until the dust, dirt are off the leaves and then rinse in salt water for about 30 minutes to kill any germs, cysts, and to rid them of any residual pesticides.

Whenever permitted, use collards while they are fresh. Collards have a relatively good shelf-life; can be stored in the refrigerator for up to four days.

Preparation:

Both stalks and leaves are edible. Tough stalks and thick leaves are trimmed using paring knife. The leaves should be chopped into smaller sections to aid quick cooking. Extensive cooking may result in loss of some amount of vitamins like folates and vitamin-C.

Collard greens blend nicely with either salads or with cooked meat or fish dishes.

Its fresh leaves can be also added when making juice with other greens, fruits and herbs.

CUCUMBERS
(*Cucumis sativus*, Linn.)

Next to tomatoes, cabbage, and onions, cucumbers are the fourth most widely cultivated vegetable in the world. They are enjoyed on virtually all continents and you will find them being incorporated into all types of cuisine.

Cucumbers are rich in water, and contain but little mineral matter; they are chiefly prized for their agreeable odor and flavor. Cooked they form an attractive and easily digested succulent vegetable. In Egypt, they are cooked in many attractive ways and are served daily in every household. As a preserve they form the common sweetmeat. Stuffed with crumbs and chopped nuts, they take the place of meat.

Cucumbers when served raw are dense and difficult of digestion; if sliced and soaked in salted water they lose their crispness, become leathery and even dangerous to persons of weak stomach. Always soak them in clear, cold water.

Even though long, dark green, smooth-skinned garden cucumbers are familiar vegetables in the produce sections of most groceries, cucumbers actually come in a wide variety of colors, sizes, shapes and textures. You'll find white, yellow, and even orange-colored cucumbers, and they may be short, slightly oval, or even round in shape. Their skins can be smooth and thin, or thick and rough. In a technical sense, cucumbers are actually fruits, not vegetables.

While there are literally hundreds of different varieties of *Cucumis sativus*, virtually all can be divided into two basic types: slicing and pickling. Slicing cucumbers include all varieties that are cultivated for consumption in fresh form.

Armenian cucumbers *(Cucumis melo var. flexuosus)* are long, crispy, and thin-ribbed, curved, and have light green color. Although grouped botanically in the melon family, they appear and taste just like cucumbers.

Miniature varieties such as **gherkins**, American-dills, and French-*cornichons* are very small indeed and usually preferred in pickling.

Dosakayi is a yellow Indian curry cucumber, has sweet taste and neutral flavor. It is used extensively in the preparation of stews and curries, particularly during the summer season in southern parts of India and Sri Lanka.

Health Benefits:

- It is one of the very low calorie vegetables; provide just 15 calories per 100 g. It contains no saturated fats or cholesterol. Cucumber peel is a good source of dietary fiber that helps reduce constipation, and offer some protection against colon cancers by eliminating toxic compounds from the gut.

- It is a very good source of potassium, an important intracellular electrolyte. Potassium is a heart friendly electrolyte helps bring a reduction in total blood pressure and heart rates by countering effects of sodium.

- Cucumbers contains unique anti-oxidants in moderate ratios such as β-carotene and α-carotene, vitamin-C, vitamin-A, *zea-xanthin* and *lutein*. These compounds help act as protective scavengers against oxygen-derived free radicals and reactive oxygen species (ROS) that play a role in aging and various disease processes.

- Cucumbers have mild diuretic property, which perhaps attributed to their free-water, and potassium and low sodium content. This helps in checking weight gain and high blood pressure.

- They surprisingly have a high amount of vitamin K. Vitamin-K has been found to have a potential role in bone strength by promoting osteotrophic (bone mass building) activity. It also has established role in the treatment of Alzheimer's disease patients by limiting neuronal damage in their brain.

Selection and storage:

Cucumbers are readily sold in the stores year around. Fresh varieties, depending upon the cultivar type and region, as well as preserved, pre-processed, and pickled are also available in stores.

In the store, buy fresh ones that feature bright green color, firm and stout in texture. Look for spots, cuts or breaks over its surface. Do not buy overly matur or yellow since they tend to contain more insoluble fiber and mature seeds. Furthermore, avoid those with wrinkled ends as they indicate old stock and state of de-hydration. Go for organically grown products to get rich flavor and nutrient content.

Once at home, they should be washed thoroughly in clean water to remove any surface dust and pesticides. The skin comes in a variety of colors and often with tiny spikes that should be rubbed off. Do not discard the peel as it has vital minerals, phyto-chemicals, and fiber.

To store, keep them at room temperature for a day or two, but better stored inside the refrigerator set at high relative humidity where they stay fresh for several days.

Preparation:

Wash them thoroughly in cold running water just before use. Sometimes, they may require light scrub at places where prickles or dirt attached firmly. Trim both ends using sharp knife and rub the ends to remove sticky, off-white, fluid like oozing substance in order to lessen bitter taste of either ends. Cut into cubes, slices, etc., as you may desire.

Fresh, clean cucumbers may be enjoyed as is.

They may be cut into cubes as a addition to vegetable or fruit salads.

The dosakayi cucumber is used in a variety of curry and stew preparations.

Finely chopped fresh slices mixed with yogurt, cumin, coriander, pepper and salt make an Indian dish called cucumber raita.

Cucumber juice is a very good health drink.

Gherkin and rind of other varieties are used in the preparation of pickles.

EGG PLANT
(*Solanum melongena*, Linn., Variety *esculentum*)

Eggplant, or *aubergine* as it is called in France, is a vegetable long prized for its beauty as well as its unique taste and texture. Eggplants belong to the plant family of *Solanaceae*, also commonly known as nightshades, and are kin to the tomato, bell pepper and potato. Eggplants grow in a manner much like tomatoes, hanging from the vines of a plant that grows several feet in height.

One of the most popular varieties of eggplant in North America looks like a pear-shaped egg, a characteristic from which its name is derived. The skin is glossy and deep purple in color, while the flesh is cream colored and spongy in consistency. Contained within the flesh are seeds arranged in a conical pattern.

In addition to this variety, eggplant is also available in a cornucopia of other colors including lavender, jade green, orange, and yellow-white, as well as in sizes and shapes that range from that of a small tomato to a large zucchini.

While the different varieties do vary slightly in taste and texture, one can generally describe the eggplant as having a pleasantly bitter taste and spongy texture. In many recipes, eggplant fulfills the role of being a complementary ingredient that balances the surrounding flavors of the other more pronounced ingredients.

In England the egg plant is called *aubergines* or *brinjal*. The large purple variety is best.

Health Benefits:
- Eggplant is very low in calories and fats but rich in soluble fiber content.
- Research studies suggested that eggplant is effective to control high blood cholesterol.
- The peel or skin (deep blue/purple varieties) of aubergine has significant amounts of phenolic flavonoid phyto-chemicals called *anthocyanins*. Scientific studies have shown that these anti-oxidants have potential health effects against

cancer, aging, inflammation, and neurological diseases.

- It contains good amounts of many essential B-complex groups of vitamins such as pantothenic acid (vitamin B5), pyridoxine (vitamin B6) and thiamin (vitamin B1), niacin (B3). These vitamins are essential in the sense that body requires them from external sources to replenish and required for fat, protein and carbohydrate metabolism.
- Further, this vegetable is an also good source of minerals like manganese, copper, iron and potassium. Manganese is used as a co-factor for the antioxidant enzyme, *superoxide dismutase*. Potassium is an important intracellular electrolyte helps counter the hypertension effects of sodium.

Selection and storage:

Eggplants are available year round. In the stores, varieties of eggplants varying in size, shape, and color are sold.

Buy healthy looking, firm, shiny, bright-colored fruits that feel heavy and solid. Take a close look at the stalk; if it is stout, firm, and green that means the fruit is fresh.

Avoid those shriveled, soft in hand and with wrinkles, surface cuts or bruise. Always avoid over-mature, old-stock, and sunken eggplants as they taste bitter and, therefore, unappetizing.

At home, they can be kept in cool place for use in a day or two but ideally should be stored inside the refrigerator set at high relative humidity, where they keep fresh for few days.

Preparation:

Wash eggplant thoroughly in cold water before use. Trim the stalk end using a sharp knife. Sprinkle a pinch of cooking salt or soak pieces in salt water to remove the bitter compounds. Whole fruit, including its skin and fine, tiny seeds are edible.

Whole, cubed, or sliced; aubergine can be used in variety of recipes

Spicy aubergine slices can be used as a side dish in salads or appetizer.

It can be stew fried, roasted, baked or ground in the preparation of a variety of recipes.

In Southern India, it is chopped into cubes and used in curry, chutney, and with rice.

A popular recipe in the Mediterranean region is stewed asparagus spears sandwiched with eggplant slices.

It is also widely used in pickling.

HORSERADISH
(*Nasturtium Arnwracia*, Fries)

Horseradish has been cultivated since antiquity. According to Greek mythology, the Delphic Oracle told Apollo that the horseradish was worth its weight in gold.

Horseradish was known in Egypt in 1500 BC. Dioscorides listed horseradish under *Thlaspi* or *Persicon*; Cato discusses the plant in his treatises on agriculture, and a mural in Pompeii shows the plant. Horseradish is probably the plant mentioned by Pliny the Elder in his Natural History under the name of *Amoracia*, and recommended by him for its medicinal qualities, and possibly the Wild Radish, or *raphanos agrios* of the Greeks. The early Renaissance herbalists Pietro Andrea Mattioli and John Gerard showed it under Raphanus.

Both root and leaves were used as a medicine during the Middle Ages and the root was used as a condiment on meats in Germany, Scandinavia, and Britain. It was brought to North America during Colonial times.[

The edible portion of this plant consists of the long tap root, which contains very much the same aromatic principles as the black mustard. This is usually grated, mixed with vinegar, and served as a condiment or sauce for cold meats, raw oysters or clams. Carefully cooked it is less pungent and much more palatable than raw, and is then served as an accompaniment to game.

KALE

The beautiful leaves of the kale plant provide an earthy flavor and more nutritional value for fewer calories than almost any other food around. Although it can be found in markets throughout the year, it is in season from the middle of winter through the beginning of spring when it has a sweeter taste and is more widely available.

Kale is distinguished from savoy by the abundance of chlorophyll, the green coloring matter of the leaves, and the short stem from which the leaves spring. Kale is the least nutritious of all the cabbage tribe. It contains very little vegetable acid and flavoring substance; it forms, however, one of the most agreeable and best of the spring greens. We have two varieties, blue and green; both are prepared precisely the same.

Health Benefits:

- Kale is a very versatile and nutritious green leafy vegetable. It is a widely popular vegetable since ancient Greek and Roman times for its low fat, no cholesterol but health benefiting anti-oxidant properties.
- Kale, like other members of the Brassica family, contains health-promoting phytochemicals, sulforaphane and indole-3-carbinol that appear to protect against prostate and colon cancers.
- Di-indolyl-methane (DIM), a metabolite of *indole-3-carbinol* is an effective immune modulator, anti-bacterial and anti-viral agent through its action of potentiating "Interferon-Gamma" receptors.
- Borecole is very rich source of β-carotene, lutein and zea-xanthin. These flavonoids have strong anti-oxidant and anti-cancer activities. Beta-carotene is converted to vitamin A in the body.

- Zea-xanthin, an important dietary carotenoid, is selectively absorbed into the retinal macula lutea in the eyes where it is thought to provide antioxidant and protective light-filtering functions. Thus, it helps prevent retinal detachment and offer protection against "age-related macular degeneration related macular degeneration disease" (ARMD) in the elderly.
- It is very rich in vitamin A. Vitamin A is required for maintaining healthy mucus membranes and skin and is essential for vision. Foods rich in this vitamin are known to offer protection against lung and oral cavity cancers.
- It is one of the excellent vegetable sources for vitamin-K. Vitamin K has potential role bone health by promoting osteotrophic (bone formation and strengthening) activity. Adequate vitamin-K levels in the diet help limiting neuronal damage in the brain; thus, has established role in the treatment of patients suffering from Alzheimer's disease.
- Kale is very rich in Vitamin C. Vitamin C is a powerful antioxidant, which helps the body develop resistance against infectious agents and scavenge harmful oxygen-free radicals.
- This leafy vegetable is notably good in many B-complex groups of vitamins such as niacin, vitamin B-6 (pyridoxine), thiamin, pantothenic

acid, etc., that are essential for substrate metabolism in the body.

- It is also rich source of minerals like copper, calcium, sodium, potassium, iron, manganese, and phosphorus. Potassium is an important component of cell and body fluids that helps controlling heart rate and blood pressure by countering effects of sodium. Manganese is used by the body as a co-factor for the antioxidant enzyme, *superoxide dismutase*. Iron is required for cellular oxidation and red blood cell formation.

Selection and storage:

Kale is available at its best during winter months from November until March. Exposure of crop to light frost, in fact, enhances its eating quality. While harvesting, individual lower leaves may be picked either progressively as the main stem elongates or the whole plant is cut at the stem and packed in bundles. In the store, buy fresh green leaves featuring crispy, crunchy, brilliant dark blue-green color.

Borecole, like chard, is an extremely perishable leafy vegetable, so should be used quickly once harvested. If at all to be stored inside the refrigerator set its temperature below 35 degree F and high humidity level to maintain vitality.

Preparation:

As in spinach, borecole should be washed thoroughly in clean running water and swished in saline water for about

10-15 minutes in order to remove soil, dirt and any fungicide/insecticide residues.

Just before cooking, remove tough stems, and separate wilted leaves from healthy ones. The leaves are generally blanched before use in cooking.

Fresh young borecole can be sued raw in salads.

Mature leaves and stalks are typically coked or sautéed.

Tuscan kale leaves are popular winter staples in Mediterranean regions, used in soups, stews, salads, pizza and pasta.

KOHL-RABI

Kohl-rabi or kale-turnip, is a cultivated variety of kale or cabbage, distinguished by the swelling of the stem, just above the ground, in a turnip form, to the size of a man's fist; the larger leaf stalks springing from the swollen part. The Kohl-rabi stores nourishment just above the ground in a these turnip-like swelling of the stem. It may be boiled and served with melted butter, but is better served uncooked in slices or fancy shapes, as an accompaniment to cold meat dishes.Being free from starch it may be pared, sliced and served raw in place of radishes. Or it may be cooked and served according to the rules for cooking turnips. It is slightly more nutritious than the common white turnips. Plain boiled with cream sauce it gives a delightful, succulent fall vegetable. It is also nice in salad.

Health Benefits:

- Mildly sweet, succulent kohlrabi is notably rich in vitamins and dietary fiber; however, it has only 27 calories per 100 g, a negligible amount of fat, and zero cholesterol.

- Fresh kohlrabi stem is rich source of *vitamin-C.* Vitamin C (ascorbic acid) is a water-soluble vitamin and powerful anti-oxidant. It helps the body maintain healthy connective tissue, teeth, and gum. Its anti-oxidant property helps the human body protect from diseases and cancers by scavenging harmful free radicals from the body.

- Kohlrabi, like other members of the Brassica family, contains health-promoting phytochemicals such as isothiocyanates, sulforaphane, and indole-3-carbinol that are supposed to protect against prostate and colon cancers.

- It especially contains good amounts of many B-complex groups of vitamins such as niacin, vitamin B-6 (pyridoxine), thiamin, pantothenic acid, etc., that acts as co-factors to enzymes during various metabolism inside the body.

- Knol-knol notably has good levels of minerals; copper, calcium, potassium, manganese, iron, and phosphorus are especially available in the stem. Potassium is an important component of cell and body fluids that helps controlling heart rate and blood pressure by countering effects of sodium.

Manganese is used by the body as a co-factor for the antioxidant enzyme, *superoxide dismutase.*

- In addition, its creamy color flesh contains small amounts of vitamin A and carotenes.
- Kohlrabi leaves or tops, like turnip greens, are also very nutritious greens abundant in carotenes, vitamin A, vitamin K, minerals, and B-complex group of vitamins.

Selection and storage:

This attractive stem vegetable is available at its best during winter months from November until March. Over maturity as well as exposure of crop to excessive sunlight makes the stem woody and tough in texture resulting in its poor eating quality. Fresh kohlrabies should have crunchy texture and impart rich flavor.

In the stores, buy medium-sized, fresh tubers and heavy in hand for their size. Avoid those with cracks, cuts, spoiled or mold infested. Do not buy if they have lighter weight for their size and excessively woody in consistency as it indicates signs of over-maturity and unappetizing.

Knol-knols exhibit good keeping qualities and can be placed at room temperature for 2-3 days. However, If you wish to store for few more days, then keep them in the refrigerator set at temperature below 35 degree F and high humidity level to maintain vitality.

Preparation:

Kohlrabi stems should be washed thoroughly in clean running water and swish in saline water for about 10-15 minutes in order to remove any surface soil, dirt and any insecticide/fungicide residues.

Just before cooking, remove any leaves and trim the stem ends. Peel the skin using paring knife.

Fresh young crispy kohlrabi can be used raw in salad/coleslaw.

It mixes well with other vegetables and greens in a variety of recipes.

Peeled stem, cut into slices or cubes, can be mixed with other vegetables like potatoes and stewed with onion, garlic and tomato.

Stewed kohlrabi cubes mix well with meats and poultry.

LEEK
(*Allium Porrum*, Linn.)

Leeks, known scientifically as *Allium porrum*, are related to garlic, onions, shallots, and scallions. Leeks look like large scallions, having a very small bulb and a long white cylindrical stalk of superimposed layers that flows into green, tightly wrapped, flat leaves. Cultivated leeks are usually about 12 inches in length and one to two inches in diameter and feature a fragrant flavor that is reminiscent of shallots but sweeter and more subtle. Wild leeks, known as ramps, are much smaller in size, but have a stronger, more intense flavor. They are available for a short period of time each year and are often widely sought out at farmers markets when they are in season.

With a more delicate and sweeter flavor than onions, leeks add a subtle touch to recipes without overpowering the other flavors that are present. Although leeks are available throughout the year they are in season from the fall through the early part of spring when they are at their best.

The flavonoids in leeks are most concentrated in their lower leaf and bulb portion. The flavonol kaempferol is one of leeks' premiere flavonoids, and it's also most concentrated in the lower leaf and bulb. Leeks rank ahead of white onions in terms of their kaempferol content, but they still provide slightly less kaempferol than red onions. For other types of flavonoids, including quercetin, leeks appear to provide lower concentrations than most types of onions.

Leeks, like garlic and onions, belong to a vegetable family called the Allium vegetables. Since leeks are related to garlic and onions, they contain many of the same beneficial compounds found in these well-researched, health-promoting vegetables.

The bulb of the leek is greatly elongated, and the leaves broadly linear. They are used principally as flavoring for soups, but are sometimes boiled and served with cream sauce.

Health Benefits:
- Leeks contain many noteworthy flavonoid anti-oxidants, minerals, and vitamins that have proven health benefits.

- Leeks are low in calories. Further, their elongated stalks provide good amounts of soluble and insoluble fiber.
- Though leeks contain proportionately less thio-sulfinites than that in garlic, they still possess significant amounts of these anti-oxidants such as *diallyl disulfide, diallyl trisulfide* and *allyl propyl disulfide*. The compounds convert to allicin by enzymatic reaction when the leek-stalk disturbed (crushing, cutting, etc).
- Laboratory studies show that *allicin* reduces cholesterol production by inhibiting the *HMG-CoA reductase* enzyme in the liver cells. Further, it also found to have anti-bacterial, anti-viral and anti-fungal activities.
- Additionally, allicin decreases blood vessel stiffness by release of nitric oxide (NO) and, thereby bring a reduction in the total blood pressure. It also blocks platelet clot formation and has fibrinolytic action in the blood vessels, which helps decrease an overall risk of coronary artery disease (CAD), peripheral vascular diseases (PVD), and stroke.
- Leeks are a great source of minerals and vitamins that are essential for optimum health. Their leafy stems indeed contain several vital vitamins such as pyridoxine, folic acid, niacin, riboflavin, and thiamin in healthy proportions. Folic acid is essential for DNA synthesis and cell division. Their

adequate levels in the diet during pregnancy can help prevent neural tube defects in the newborn babies.

- In addition, leeks are one of the good sources of vitamin-A and other flavonoid phenolic anti-oxidants such as carotenes, xanthin, and lutein. They also have some other essential vitamins such as vitamin C, K, and vitamin E. Vitamin C helps the human body develop resistance against infectious agents and scavenge harmful, pro-inflammatory free radicals.

- Further, its stalks have small amounts of minerals such as potassium, iron, calcium, magnesium, manganese, zinc, and selenium.

Selection and storage:

Leeks are at their best during spring season. However, they can be available fresh year around in most of the super markets. While buying, choose fresh organic leeks, as they are rich in flavor and in nutrition. Look for uniform, long, firm, white stalks with healthy root bulb as it signals of fresh farm produce.

Avoid stems with withered, yellow discolor tops.

Once at home, wrap in a paper towel and place inside the refrigerator where they stay fresh for up to a week or so.

Preparation:

Leeks impart a mellow, sweet onion-flavor to the dishes they added to. They give less pungency than garlic or onions.

Although used sparingly outside the European continent, their delicate stems have recently found favor among oriental and Mediterranean recipes.

To prepare; remove its thick top greens. Similarly, trim away lower root end. In a large bowl of water, swish the stalk gently to remove any surface grit, sand, and soil. Drain and mop dry using a paper towel.

Peel their outer layers by hand. You may want to cut them into rings, slice lengthwise or in squares using knife depending up on recipes.

Sliced baby leeks and young tender regular stem can be used raw in salads.

They mix well especially with vegetables, cream, butter, cheese, seafood, and eggs.

Delicate stems are one of the most sought after particularly in stews and soups. Potato-leek soup is a favorite Northern European winter dish.

Julienned blanch leeks are used in the preparation of quiche.

The old and popular dish, cock-a-leekie, a chicken soup, is thickened with leeks.

MARTYNIA
(*Martynia prohoscidea*, Clox.)

These plants are grown for their curious fruits, which are used principally for pickling. Containing mucilage as they do, they are in many places substituted for okra. They may be cooked and served according to the rules for cooking okra; they are not, however, so palatable.

MORINGA

Moringa oleifera, known popularly as *drumstick tree*, is an herbaceous plant grown for its nutritious greens, flowers, and mineral-rich pods. It is a well-recognized member in the *Moringaceae* family of trees and thought to be originated in the sub-Himalayan ranges of Indian subcontinent. The plant possesses horseradish-like root and, hence, known to the western world as horseradish tree. The seed pods are popular as *murnga* in Tamil, and *malunggay* in Philippines.

Moringa is a drought tolerant, medium-sized, evergreen tree that prefers warm, frost-free climates to flourish. Its tender leaves and twigs can be harvested from a well-established, 1.5 to 2 meters height plant. Taller plants bear cream-white color small size flowers in clusters throughout the season, which subsequently develop to long slender dark-green color, three-sided, edible seedpods with tapering ends. Each pod measures about 6-18 inches in length, with constrictions at the seed nodes giving them a typical drumstick appearance. Inside, each pod features fleshy pulp and round pea-sized seeds encased in a wing-shaped coat (hull).

Health Benefits:
- Moringa plant possesses unique nutritional qualities that hold promise to millions of

impoverished communities around the world. Those that lack in many nutritional supplements such as protein, minerals, and vitamins.

- Leaves are an excellent source of protein that can be rarely found in any other herbs and green leafy vegetables. Dry, powdered leaves indeed are a much-concentrated source of many quality amino acids.

- Fresh pods and seeds are a good source of oleic acid, a health-benefiting monounsaturated fat. Moringa as high-quality oilseed crop can be grown alternatively to improve nutrition levels of populations in many drought-prone regions of Africa and Asia.

- Fresh leaves and growing tips of moringa are the richest source of vitamin A. Vitamin A is one of the fat-soluble anti-oxidant offering several benefits, including mucus membrane repair, maintenance of skin integrity, vision, and immunity.

- Fresh moringa pods and leaves are excellent sources of vitamin-C. Research studies have shown that consumption of fruits/vegetables rich in vitamin C helps the body develop immunity against infectious agents, and scavenge harmful oxygen-free radicals from the body.

- The greens as well as pods also contain good amounts of many vital B-complex vitamins such as folates, vitamin-B6 (pyridoxine), thiamin (vitamin B-1), riboflavin, pantothenic acid, and niacin.

Much of these vitamin functions as co-enzymes in carbohydrate, protein, and fat metabolism.

- Furthermore, its leaves are one of the fine sources of minerals like calcium, iron, copper, manganese, zinc, selenium, and magnesium. Iron alleviates anemia. Calcium is required for bone strengthening. Zinc plays a vital role in hair-growth, spermatogenesis, and skin health.

Selection and storage:

Fresh moringa pods and greens are readily available in the markets all around the season in the tropical and sub-tropical countries of South-East Asia, Philippines, Middle-Eastern, Africa, Caribbean, and in some Central American region. In the USA, The tree grows easily in the Southern states; however, only few owners grow them in their backyard. Its consumption in the USA is mainly driven by several thousand expatriated communities of Asian and African background, who prefer the M.oleifera plant parts in their diet.

Fresh leaves, pods, seed-kernels as well as dry powder, canned, etc. can be found in some specialized stores. At their nativity, moringa leaves are one of the inexpensive greens available in the markets. However, fresh pods and seeds command good price even in the native Asian and African markets.

While buying fresh pods look for just tender, uniform, evenly filled, green color pods. Avoid dry, shriveled, bent, twisted, or broken pods. Do not by over-mature big size pods as they feature tougher skin, bitter pulp and hard seeds and thus unappetizing.

At home, greens should be stored as in other greens. Pods can keep well for 1-2 days at room temperature, however, should be kept in the refrigerator for extended shelf life.

Dried moringa leaf powder and capsules are also sold in the stores for their advocated health-benefits across Europe and North Americas.

Preparation:

Fresh greens and tender seedpods are used extensively in the cooking in Asia, Africa and Caribbean cuisine. Only tender growing tips and young leaves are generally used as greens in the cooking. However, mature leaves are dried, powdered and can be stored for longer periods to be used in the recipes.

Clean and wash the greens in cold water as you do in case of other greens like spinach. To prepare fresh pods, clean them in cold water and mop dry using an absorbent paper towel. Trim the ends. Cut the pod at one to two inches intervals and use in soups, curries, etc. Clean the leaves as you do for other greens like fenugreek, purslane, spinach, etc. Sift the leaves from the twig and discard the stem. Chop the leaves if you wish, otherwise, its whole leaves can be used in the recipes.

Morning pods and greens are used regularly in many Asian traditions. In the Philippines, where they are available year around, its leaves are used in soups, stews with fish, prawns, and poultry.

In traditional Senegalese recipe, moringa green are used to prepare a sauce. Fresh leaves are sautéed with onion, peanut butter, vegetable oil, smoked-dried fish, and seasoned with salt and pepper.

In South Indian states, both pods and greens are used in curries, soups, and stews.

Dry and powdered moringa, leaves can be added to diet in order to improve the nutritional quality in Africa and Asia.

OKRA
(*Hibiscus esculentus*, Linn.)

Okra, also known as *"lady finger"* is one of the highly nutritious vegetables, usually eaten while the pod is green, tender, and immature. Botanically, this perennial flowering plant belongs to the Malvaceae *(mallows)* family and named scientifically as Abelmoschus esculentus.

The plant is cultivated throughout the tropical and warm temperate regions around the world for its fibrous fruits or "pods." It grows best in well-drained and manure rich soil. The plant bears numerous dark green colored pods measuring about 5-15 cm in length. It takes about 45-60 days to get ready-to-harvest fruits.

Internally, the pods feature small, round, mucilaginous white colored seeds arranged in vertical rows. The pods are handpicked while just short of reaching maturity and eaten as a vegetable.

The young pods constitute the edible portion of this plant. They are rich in mucilage and used principally for soups. The Creoles use them with corn and tomatoes as a stew, and with tomatoes alone as a sauce. They form the base of all varieties of gumbo. The famous Brunswick stew of Virginia is a sort of gumbo. Okra may be preserved for winter use by cutting them into rings, stringing them on cords and drying in the hot air; or they may be canned the same as other vegetables. Okra is frequently called gumbo.

Health Benefits:

- The pods are among the very low calorie vegetables and containing no saturated fats or cholesterol. Nonetheless, they are rich sources of dietary fiber, minerals, and vitamins; often recommended by nutritionists in cholesterol controlling and weight reduction programs.
- The rich fiber and *mucilaginous* content in okra pods help in smooth peristalsis of digested food particles and relieve constipation condition.
- The pods contain healthy amounts of vitamin A, and flavonoid anti-oxidants such as beta carotenes, xanthin and lutein. It is one of the *green* vegetables with highest levels of these anti-oxidants. These compounds are known to have antioxidant properties and are essential for vision. Vitamin A is also required for maintaining healthy mucus membranes and skin. Consumption of

natural vegetables and fruits rich in flavonoids helps to protect from lung and oral cavity cancers.

- Fresh pods are the good source of folates. Consumption of foods rich in folates, especially during the pre-conception period helps decrease the incidence of neural tube defects in the offspring.

- The gumbo pods are also an excellent source of anti-oxidant vitamin, vitamin-C. Research suggests that consumption of foods rich in vitamin-C helps the body develop immunity against infectious agents, reduce episodes of cold and cough and protect the body from harmful free radicals.

- The veggies are rich in B-complex group of vitamins like niacin, vitamin B-6 (pyridoxine), thiamin and pantothenic acid. The pods also contain good amounts of vitamin K. Vitamin K is a co-factor for blood clotting enzymes and is required for strengthening of bones.

- The pods are an also good source of many important minerals such as iron, calcium, manganese and magnesium.

Selection and storage:

Fresh and immature okra pods are readily available in the stores all around the year. The pods feature attractively rich green-color and have neutral flavor. In the store, look for crispy, immature pods and avoid those with over-ripen, sunken appearance, discolored spots, cuts and too soft.

Once at home, place them inside the refrigerator. Eat them while they are fresh to obtain full benefits of vitamins and anti-oxidants.

Preparation:

In general, some of the hybrid varieties are subject to insecticide/pesticide spray. Therefore, wash the pods thoroughly in the water in order to remove dust, soil and any residual insecticides.

Trim the top stem end using a paring knife. Some prefer trimming tip ends as well. Then, cut/slice the pod as desired.

Okra pods are one of the widely used vegetables in tropical countries. Chopped of sliced pods are stewed or fried under low heat oil in order to soften. They then can be mixed with other vegetables, rice, or meat.

In Caribbean islands, okra is cooked and eaten as soup, often with fish.

The pods can be pickled and preserved like other vegetables.

Okra leaves may be cooked in a similar manner as the greens of beets or dandelions. The leaves are also eaten raw in salads.

ONION
(*Allium Cepa*, Linn.)

The common onion consists of a large bulb containing very pungent flavoring due to a volatile oil rich in sulphur. This odor, like the odor of cabbage, is dissipated and thrown off by careless cooking. Onions must be cooked in salted boiling water, in an uncovered vessel; they are then wholesome, rather easy of digestion and stimulating to the intestines.

Varieties differ in containing more or less volatile oil. The Spanish and Bermuda onions contain but little and are termed "sweet," while our common "brown skins" are very pungent.

To keep for winter use, select a perfectly light, dry place where there is no danger of the onions freezing — they must be kept cold, but freezing causes immediate decay. Too warm a place causes sprouting. A temperature of 50° Fahr. is about right.

Onions, like garlic, are members of the Allium family, and both are rich in sulfur-containing compounds that are responsible for their pungent odors and for many of their health-promoting effects.

Health Benefits:
- Onions are very low in calories and fats; however, rich in soluble dietary fiber.
- Phyto-chemical compounds *allium* and *Allyl disulphide* in the onion convert to *allicin* by

176

enzymatic reaction when its modified leaves are distorted (crushing, cutting, etc.). Studies have shown that these compounds have anti-mutagenic (protects from cancers) and anti-diabetic properties (helps lower blood sugar levels in diabetics).

- Laboratory studies show that *allicin* reduces cholesterol production by inhibiting the *HMG-CoA reductase* enzyme in the liver cells. Further, it also found to have anti-bacterial, anti-viral, and anti-fungal activities.

- In addition, *Allicin* also decreases blood vessel stiffness by releasing nitric oxide (NO) and thereby bring a reduction in the total blood pressure. Further, it blocks platelet-clot formation and has fibrinolytic action in the blood vessels. Altogether, it helps decrease an overall risk of coronary artery disease (CAD), peripheral vascular diseases (PVD), and stroke.

- Onions are rich source of chromium, the trace mineral that helps tissue cells respond appropriately to insulin levels in the blood. It thus helps facilitate insulin action and control sugar levels in diabetes.

- They are an also good source of antioxidant flavonoid *quercetin*, which is found to have anti-carcinogenic, anti-inflammatory, and anti-diabetic functions.

- They are also good in antioxidant vitamin, vitamin-C and mineral manganese. Manganese is required as a co-factor for anti-oxidant enzyme, *superoxide dismutase.* In addition, *isothiocyanate* anti-oxidants in them help provide relief from cold and flu by exerting anti-inflammatory actions.
- Onions are also good in B-complex group of vitamins like pantothenic acid, pyridoxine, folates and thiamin. Pyridoxine or vitamin B-6 helps keep up GABA levels in the brain, which works against neurotic conditions.

Selection and storage:

Raw onions are readily available during all the seasons. Depending on the variety, they can be sharp, spicy, tangy and pungent or mild and sweet. In the store, they are available in fresh, frozen, canned, pickled, powdered, and dehydrated forms.

While buying, look for fresh ones that are clean, well shaped, have no opening at the neck and feature crispy, and dry outer skins. Avoid those that show sprouting or have signs of black mold (a kind of fungal attack) as they indicate that the stock is old. In addition, poor-quality bulbs often have soft spots, moisture at their neck, and dark patches, which may all be indications of decay.

At home, store them in cool dark place away from moisture and humid conditions where they keep fresh for several days. They can also keep well in the refrigerator; however, you should use them immediately once you remove from the refrigerator since they tend to spoil if they kept at room temperature for a while.

Preparation:

Trim the ends using a sharp knife. Then peel the outer 2-3 layers of skin until you find fresh thick pinkish-white whorls. You can slice or cut them into fine cubes depending upon the recipe type. Top greens and flower heads are also edible. Spring onions or *scallions* are favored in fast food preparations.

They are used either chopped or sliced, in almost every type of food, including fresh salads, or as a spicy garnish.

In India and Pakistan, onions are one of the most sought-after ingredients in cooking where they used in curries, stir-fries, soups, stuffing, pastes, sauces, etc.

They are one of the common ingredients in the Chinese "chowmein".

They are used extensively in Mediterranean and continental cooking in salads, cheese pizza, soup, rolls, stuffing, etc.

Safety Precaution:

Raw onions can cause irritation to skin, mucus membranes and eyes. Its effect can be minimized by immersing the trimmed bulb in cold water for a few minutes before you chop or slice it.

PEPPERS
(CHILLIES)

The very many diverse forms of "peppers" are obtained from the varieties of two or three species of the genus *Capsicum*, the commonest of which is *Capsicum annuum*, Linn. Tobasco and the best cayenne are made from the small yellow, red, very hot or pungent "bird pepper." Paprika is made from a brilliant red, sweet chilli, dried and ground. This is used as a coloring and flavoring for sauces, soups and salads.

The large sweet varieties, stuffed or stewed, form an agreeable succulent vegetable. The large hot chillies or "bell" peppers are used principally by the Mexicans as a base or flavoring for all made dishes, as tamales and chile-con-carne. They are used by Americans stuffed with cabbage, and pickled, as mangoes.

Tobasco oil is made by soaking "bird peppers" in olive oil. It forms an exceedingly pleasant seasoning for cream sauce or salad dressings. Sweet chillies are canned or dried, for winter use. If dried they must be soaked in water before cooking. A very nice Spanish pepper, canned in oil, can be purchased at any first-class grocer's. These are used as a salad garnish, or as a seasoning for oysters or stewed chicken.

It's not surprising that chili peppers can trace their history to Central and South America, regions whose cuisines are renowned for their hot and spicy flavors. Chili peppers have been cultivated in these regions for more than seven thousand years, first as a decorative item and later as a foodstuff and medicine.

It was not until the 15th and 16th centuries that chili peppers were introduced to the rest of the world. Christopher Columbus encountered them on his explorations of the Caribbean Islands and brought them back to Europe. There, they were used as a substitute for black pepper, which was very expensive since it had to be imported from Asia.

There are hundreds of different types of chili peppers that vary in size, shape, color, flavor and "hotness." This fleshy berry features many seeds inside a potent package that can range from less than one inch to six inches in length, and approximately one-half to one inch in diameter. Chili peppers are usually red or green in color.

Chili peppers have many health benefits including fighting inflammation; natural pain relief; cardiovascular benefits; clear congestion; boost immunity; helps stop the spread of prostate cancer; prevents stomach ulcers; lose weight; and lowers risk of type 2 diabetes.

Health Benefits:
- Bell pepper contains an impressive list of plant nutrients that are known to have disease preventing and health promoting properties. Unlike other chili peppers, it is very low in calories and fats. 100 g provide just 31 calories.
- Sweet (bell) pepper contains small levels of health benefiting an alkaloid compound capsaicin. Early laboratory studies on experimental mammals

suggest that capsaicin has anti-bacterial, anti-carcinogenic, analgesic and anti-diabetic properties. When used judiciously, it also found to reduce triglycerides and LDL cholesterol levels in obese individuals.

- Fresh bell peppers, red or green, are rich source of vitamin-C. This vitamin is especially concentrated in red peppers at highest levels. Vitamin-C is a potent water soluble antioxidant. Regular consumption of foods rich in this vitamin helps the human body protect from scurvy; develop resistance against infectious agents (boosts immunity) and scavenge harmful, pro-inflammatory free radicals from the body.

- It also contains good levels of vitamin-A. In addition, it contains anti-oxidant flavonoids such as α and β carotenes, lutein, zea-xanthin, and cryptoxanthin. Together, these antioxidant substances in capsicum help to protect the body from injurious effects of free radicals generated during stress and disease conditions.

- Bell pepper has adequate levels of essential minerals. Some of the main minerals in it are iron, copper, zinc, potassium, manganese, magnesium, and selenium. Manganese is used by the body as a co-factor for the antioxidant enzyme, superoxide dismutase. Selenium is an anti-oxidant micro-mineral that acts as a co-factor for enzyme, *superoxide dismutase*.

- Further, capsicum (sweet pepper) is also good in B-complex group of vitamins such as niacin, pyridoxine (vitamin B-6), riboflavin, and thiamin (vitamin B-1). These vitamins are essential in the sense that body requires them from external sources to replenish. B-complex vitamins facilitate cellular metabolism through various enzymatic functions.

Selection and storage:

In general, fresh bell peppers are treated like any other vegetables in the kitchen. Their firm, crunchy consistency together with delicate sweet flavor makes them one of the most sought-after vegetable items in cooking.

Avoid excessively soft, lusterless, pale green color peppers. Furthermore, avoid those with surface cuts/punctures, bruise, spots and shriveled stems.

Once at home, should be stored in the refrigerator in a plastic bag where they will stay fresh for about a 4days. If stored for prolonged periods, they may sustain the chill injuries.

Preparation:

In general, fresh bell peppers are treated like any other vegetables in the kitchen. Their firm, crunchy consistency together with delicate sweet flavor makes them one of the most sought after vegetable item in cooking.

To prepare, wash bell peppers in cold running water. Cut the stem end and discard it. Remove the central core with seeds. Chop it using paring knife into rings or strips.

Although sweet peppers have less capsaicin than chili peppers, still they may inflict burning sensation to hands and may cause irritation to mouth/nasal passages, eyes and throat. Therefore, it may be advised in some sensitive individuals to use thin hand gloves and face masks while handling.

Fresh raw bell peppers can be used as other vegetables. They can be eaten as salads or cooked in stir-fries.

In many parts of South Asia, they are mixed with other vegetables and spices in stir-fries.

They can be stuffed with rice, meat, cheese, etc., and cooked.

They can also be grilled and served with sauce, cheese, and olive oil.

RADISH
(*Raphanus sativtis*, Linn.)

Radishes contain neither sugar nor starch and are as a rule served raw as appetizers. They are passed with the soup at dinner and are frequently served for breakfast or lunch, passed at the early part of the meal. Being dense, they are rather difficult of digestion, and do not contain nourishment. Many varieties are cultivated, and when young, tender and full grown, are crisp and palatable. They should never be eaten when old or pithy; in this condition they frequently produce acute indigestion.

Daikon or Japanese radishes are native to Asia. They are generally grown during winter months and have elongated smooth, icy-white roots.

Black Spanish radishes are peppery and more flavorful than their white counterparts.

Green radish is native to Northern China region. Its outer peel near the top stem end features leafy-green color which, gradually changes to white color near the lower tip. Inside, its flesh has beautiful jade green color, sweet and less pungent flavor.

Watermelon radishes have watermelon like flesh inside. However, they taste sweet and less peppery, something similar to that of white varieties.

The small red button radishes should not be peeled or pared; the skin aids in the digestion of the radish. The tiny green seed pods are pickled and used as a garnish for salads and are one of the ingredients of mixed pickles.

The large Japanese and the solid black Spanish radishes are grown for winter use. If covered with sand in a cool cellar they will keep in good condition until spring. They may be served either raw or cooked, and if properly kept give variety to the winter dinner. Containing neither starch nor sugar, they may, when cooked, be added to the list of diabetic foods. Prepare and cook according to the recipes given for turnips.

Winter radishes may be simply pared, cut in quarters, and arranged neatly on a pretty shallow dish. Red radishes of the spring should have the roots neatly trimmed, half the top cut and trimmed, leaving little holders at the top. These may be arranged neatly in a glass dish, and served with cracked ice.

The round white radishes and the little button radishes may be served as follows: Cut off the roots close to the radish, then the tops about one inch from the radish, wash clean in cold water, then take a radish in the left hand, holding it by the top. Cut the skin from the top downwards, in several parts, as you cut an orange to remove the skin in sections, but do not detach the skin. Now run the point of the penknife under each little section of skin and loosen it down to the stem of the radish. Throw each radish as finished into a bowl of cold water. After a little practice this operation will be comparatively easy and the radishes will look more like tulips than like ordinary table radishes. Serve in a pretty dish with cracked ice, or use as a garnish for fish cutlets, lobster cutlets, breaded chops, etc. The skin of the radish should be eaten with the flesh, as it contains a substance that helps digest the radish itself.

Health Benefits:
- Since ancient times, Chinese believe that eating radish and other brassica group vegetables such as cabbage, cauliflower, and napa would immensely benefit overall health.
- They are one of very low calorie root vegetables. They are a very good source of anti-oxidants, electrolytes, minerals, vitamins and dietary fiber.
- Radish, like other cruciferous and Brassica family vegetables, contains *isothiocyanate* anti-oxidant

compound called sulforaphane. Studies suggest that sulforaphane has proven role against prostate, breast, colon and ovarian cancers by virtue of its cancer-cell growth inhibition, and cyto-toxic effects on cancer cells.

- Fresh roots are rich in vitamin C. Vitamin C is a powerful water soluble anti-oxidant required by the body for synthesis of collagen. Vitamin C helps the body scavenge harmful free radicals, prevention from cancers, inflammation and help boost immunity.

- In addition, they contain adequate levels of folates, vitamin B-6, riboflavin, thiamin and minerals such as iron, magnesium, copper and calcium.

- Further, they contain many phytochemicals like *indoles* which are detoxifying agents and zea-xanthin, lutein and beta carotene, which are flavonoid antioxidants.

Selection and storage:

In general, radishes are available year-around with peak season during winter and spring. Daikons are most flavorful and juicy during winter.

Look for roots that feature fresh, stout and firm in texture. Their top greens also should be fresh, and feature crispy green without any yellow, shriveled leaves. Avoid roots that have cracks or cuts on their surface. Look carefully for the change in their texture and color. Yellowness indicated the stock is old. If the root yields to pressure and soft, the interior likely be pithy instead of crispy.

Once at home, remove the top greens as they rob nutrients of the roots. Then wash thoroughly in clean water to rid off surface dust and soil. Store them in a zip pouch or plastic bag in the refrigerator where they remain fresh for up to a week.

Preparation:

Both root and top greens are used for cooking. Peeling may be avoided as the anti-oxidant allyl-isothiocyanates, which gives a peppery pungent flavor to radish, are thickly concentrated in the peel. Just wash the root thoroughly, trim the tip ends, and if you have to peel, then gently pare away superficial thin layer only.

Radishes re eaten raw either as a whole or as slaw or in salads with carrots, beets, cucumber, lettuce, etc.

French breakfast radishes are served with sweet-butter and salt.

The roots are mixed with other vegetables in the preparation of steamed, stir fried or sautéed recipes in many regions.

In North India and Pakistan, the root is greated and mixed with spice and seasonings and stuffed inside bread.

Radish pods are eaten raw in salads or in stirofries in many parts of Asia.

188

Its top greens oftentimes mixed with other greens like spinach, turnip-greens, etc., used in the preparation of soups, curries as well as in cooked vegetable recieps.

TO SERVE RADISHES RAW

Wash thoroughly in cold water; trim the tops, but not close to the radish, leaving one long leaf as a sort of handle. Throw them into ice or very cold water for one hour, and serve with chopped ice in an oblong or round pickle dish. If spring radishes are pared and thrown into cold water, they lose their flavor and quickly sour. The large winter radishes should be peeled and cut into thin slices, lengthwise. If eaten raw they must be thoroughly masticated.

Safety Precaution:

Radishes may contain goitrogens, plant-based compounds found in *cruciferous* and *Brassica* family vegetables like cauliflower, broccoli, etc. Goitrogens may cause swelling of thyroid gland and should be avoided in individuals with thyroid dysfunction. Healthy person should not have any problem eating.

RHUBARB

Rhubarb is usually considered to be a vegetable; however, in the United States, a New York court decided in 1947 that since it was used in the United States as a fruit, it was to be counted as a fruit for the purposes of regulations and duties.

A side effect was a reduction on imported rhubarb tariffs, as tariffs were higher for vegetables than fruits.

Rhubarb is a perennial vegetable grown for its attractive succulent rose red color edible leafy stalks. This cool-season herbaceous plant is native to Siberia and popular in many regions of Europe and North America as "pie plant." In its natural habitat, the plant expands over the ground surface as a large spread.

Rhubarb is easy to grow and lives for many years (10-15 years) once established. The plant is usually propagated by dividing the old rhizomes (roots). Well grown plant features broad heart shaped dark-green leaves with 12 to 18 inches long leaf-petioles. It is these stalks, which are used, and their top greens discarded, as they are unfit for human consumption. Usually its stalks can be harvested from second year onwards after planting when the foliage spread and stalks reached sufficient girth of about one to two inches thick.

Health Benefits:

- Rhubarb is one of the least calorie vegetables. Nonetheless, it contains some vital phyto-nutrients such as dietary fiber, poly-phenolic anti-oxidants, minerals, and vitamins. Further, its petioles contain no saturated fats or cholesterol.
- The stalks are rich in several B-complex vitamins such as folates, riboflavin, niacin, vitamin B-6 (pyridoxine), thiamin, and pantothenic acid.

- Red color stalks contain more vitamin A than in the green varieties. Further, the stalks also contain small amounts of poly-phenolic flavonoid compounds like β-carotene, zea xanthin, and lutein. These compounds convert to vitamin A inside the body and deliver same protective effects of vitamin A on the body. Vitamin A is a powerful natural anti-oxidant and is required by the body for maintaining the integrity of skin and mucus membranes. It is also an essential vitamin for healthy eye-sight. Research studies suggest that natural foods rich in vitamin A help the body protects against lung and oral cavity cancers.

- As in other greens like kale, spinach, etc., rhubarb stalks also provide good amounts of vitamin-K. Adequate vitamin-K levels in the diet help limiting neuronal damage in the brain; thus, has established role in the treatment of Alzheimer's disease.

- Its stalks also contain healthy levels of minerals like iron, copper, calcium, potassium, and phosphorus. However, most of these minerals do not absorb into the body as they are subject to chelating into insoluble complexes by oxalic acid, and excreted out from the body.

Selection and storage:

Fresh rhubarb stalks are readily available in the markets from April until August. If you are growing them in the backyard, harvest them by grabbing the base of the leaf petiole (stalk), simultaneously pull and twist as you do it while shearing celery stalks. Immediately separate the petiole from the leaf part (leaf blade). Green tops of rhubarb contain oxalic acid as well as poisonous glycosides. In addition, greens drain away nutrients from the stalk.

While buying from the markets buy fresh, firm, crispy bright-red color stalks. They usually put for sale in bunches along with other common greens. Avoid those with dull, slump or bruise or blemishes on the surface.

Once at home, harvested or purchased stalks should be placed in a plastic bag and stored inside the refrigerator set at 32°F and 95 percent relative humidity. This way, the stalks stay fresh for about 2-3 weeks.

In the shops, one may also find ready to use, processed rhubarb preparations like canned, freeze-dried form...etc.

Preparation:

Fresh rhubarb stalks a have rich sweet-tart flavor. In general, petioles of young crinkled leaf tops have less or no strings and have the sweet flavor.

To prepare: trim the ends using paring knife. Wash them in cold running water, gently scrubbing the surface using fingers. Cut stalks into 1/2-inch to 1-inch pieces using paring knife. Usually their extreme tartness is somewhat tamed by addition of sugar, honey, syrups...etc.

Its crispy, juicy stalks can be used in the preparations of sauces, preserves, jellies, jams, syrups, sorbet, juice, etc.

Rhubarb is well remembered for its delicious pies.

It can also be used in the preparations of tarts, puddings, crumbs, pancakes, muffins, strudel, etc.

Safety Precaution:

Top green part of rhubarb leaf (blade) contains unusually high amounts of oxalic acid, a naturally-occurring substance found in some vegetables. Oxalate can cause severe symptoms even at much lower concentrations than this on the human body. Symptoms may include burning in the eyes, mouth, and throat; skin edema, difficulty breathing. In severe cases, it can result in kidney failure, convulsions, coma, and death

RUTA- BAGA

Considered to be a mix between a turnip and wild cabbage, rutabagas look like yellow turnips but have a stronger flavor. They're a member of the brassica, or cabbage family, however you'll also hear them called cruciferous vegetables because they were originally named after their cross-shaped flowers. The root can be thinly sliced and eaten raw, roasted, boiled or mashed with potatoes.

Ruta-bagas may be cooked the same as common white

turnips. They are exceedingly nice browned to serve with ducks or geese.

SAVOY

Savoy (*Borecole*), a variety of common cabbage with a loose head composed of very curly or wrinkled leaves. It is rather more delicate than the ordinary cabbage and is essentially a fall or early winter cabbage. After the head is scalded and opened it looks very much like a huge rose; the leaves never become white or bleached. On account of the looseness of the head it is usually served stuffed with other materials. The separate leaves are used with Egyptian rolls, a little roll of lentils and rice.

SPINACH
(*Spinacia olcracea*, Miller)

Calorie for calorie, leafy green vegetables like spinach with its delicate texture and jade green color provide more nutrients than any other food. Although spinach is available throughout the year, its season runs from March through May and from September through October when it is the freshest, has the best flavor, and is most readily available. Spinach belongs to the same family (*Amaranthaceae-Chenopodiaceae*) as Swiss chard and beets and has the scientific name, *Spinacia oleracea*. It shares a similar taste profile with these two other vegetables, having the bitterness of beet greens and the slightly salty flavor of Swiss chard.

This name includes a number of varieties of the same plant which do not differ chemically, and may be cooked and served according to the same recipes.

Health Benefits:
- Spinach is a store house for many phyto-nutrients that have health promotional and disease prevention properties.
- It is very low in calories and. It contains a good amount of soluble dietary fiber; no wonder green spinach is one of the finest vegetable sources recommended in cholesterol controlling and weight reduction programs!
- 100 g of fresh spinach contains about 25% of daily intake of iron; one of the richest among green leafy vegetables. Iron is an important trace element required by the body for red blood cell production and as a co-factor for oxidation-reduction enzyme, *cytochrome-oxidase* during the cellular metabolism.
- Fresh leaves are rich source of several vital anti-oxidant vitamins like vitamin A, vitamin C, and flavonoid poly phenolic antioxidants such as lutein, zea-xanthin and beta-carotene. Together these compounds help act as protective scavengers against oxygen-derived free radicals and reactive

oxygen species (ROS) that play a healing role in aging and various disease processes.

- *Zea-xanthin*, an important dietary carotenoid, is selectively absorbed into the retinal macula lutea in the eyes where it is thought to provide antioxidant and protective light-filtering functions. It thus helps protect from "age-related macular related macular disease" (ARMD), especially in the elderly.

- In addition, vitamin A is required for maintaining healthy mucus membranes and skin and is essential for normal eye-sight. Consumption of natural vegetables and fruits rich in vitamin A and flavonoids also known to help the body protect from lung and oral cavity cancers.

- Spinach leaves are an excellent source of vitamin K. Vitamin K plays a vital role in strengthening the bone mass by promoting osteotrophic (bone building) activity in the bone. Additionally, it also has established role in patients with*Alzheimer's disease* by limiting neuronal damage in the brain.

- This green leafy vegetable also contains good amounts of many B-complex vitamins such as vitamin-B6(pyridoxine), thiamin (vitamin B-1), riboflavin, folates and niacin. Folates help prevent neural tube defects in the offspring.

- 100 g of farm fresh spinach has 47% of daily recommended levels of *vitamin C*. Vitamin C is a powerful antioxidant, which helps the body develop resistance against infectious agents and scavenge harmful oxygen-free radicals.

- Its leaves also contain a good amount of minerals like *potassium*, manganese, magnesium, copper and zinc. Potassium is an important component of cell and body fluids that helps controlling heart rate and blood pressure. Manganese and copper are used by the body as a co-factor for the antioxidant enzyme,*superoxide dismutase*. Copper is required in the production of red blood cells. Zinc is a co-factor in many enzymes that regulate growth and development, sperm generation, digestion and nucleic acid synthesis.
- It is also rich source of omega-3 fatty acids.

Regular consumption of spinach in the diet helps prevent osteoporosis (weakness of bones), iron-deficiency anemia. Besides, it is believed to protect the body from cardiovascular diseases and cancers of colon and prostate.

Selection and storage:

Spinach is best available during winter months. In the markets, buy fresh leaves featuring dark-green color, vitality and crispiness. Avoid those with dull/sunken leaves, yellow discoloration and spots.

Once at home, wash leaves thoroughly in clean running water and they should be rinsed in salt water for about 30 minutes in order to remove dust, insecticide residues.

Although it can be stored inside the refrigerator for up to a week, fresh leaves should be eaten at the earliest in order to get maximum nutrition benefits.

Preparation:

Wash leaves in cold water before use. Gently pat them dry using tissue or soft cloth. Trim away tough stems. Raw leaves can be either chopped, or used as they are in variety of recipes.

Fresh spinach is eaten raw either in salad, vegetable burgers, in smoothies or as juice. Antioxidant properties may decrease significantly on steaming, frying and boiling for longer periods.

Along with other vegetables, its leaves are used in the preparation of noodles, pie, pasta, rice preparations, and soups as well as in the preparation of baby-fods.

Safety Precaution:

- Reheating of spinach left-over may cause conversion of nitrates into nitrites and nitrosamines by certain bacteria that thrive on pre-prepared nitrate-rich foods, such as spinach and many other green vegetables. These poisonous compounds may be harmful to health, especially in children.

- Phytates and dietary fiber present in the leaves may interfere with the bio-availability of iron, calcium and magnesium.
- Because of its high vitamin K content, patients taking anti-coagulants such as "warfarin" are encouraged to avoid spinach in their food since it interferes with drug metabolism.
- Spinach contains oxalic acid, a naturally-occurring substance found in some vegetables, which may crystallize as oxalate stones in the urinary tract in some people. People with known oxalate urinary tract stones are advised to avoid eating certain vegetables belonging to Amaranthaceae and Brassica family. Adequate intake of water is therefore advised to maintain normal urine output.

STACHYS

(Stachys tuberosa)

The small tubers of this plant resemble, in texture and composition, the Jerusalem artichoke, and may be cooked according to the same rules. Being very small, they require but ten minutes for cooking; if overdone they are heavy and unpalatable. The shape of the tubers is that of a corkscrew, which makes them an attractive garnish for made dishes and salads.

SUMMER SQUASH
(CYMLIN)

This belongs to the pumpkin tribe. In composition, however, it more closely resembles cucumbers and vegetable marrow. When carefully cooked, it forms a delicate, easily digested, succulent vegetable. Its nutritive value is low; it simply gives variety to the daily bills of fare. It may be cooked and served according to recipes given for cucumbers. They are very nice stuffed and baked. Do not pare them for baking.

It was that long ago when domestication of summer squash originated in Mexico and Central America. Cultivation of squashes (including summer squash) quickly became popular in North, Central, and South America, and Native Americans often referred to squashes as one of the "three sisters" alongside of corn (maize) and beans. Squashes were one of the North American foods that Columbus brought back to Spain from North America, and Portuguese and Spanish explorers introduced squashes to many parts of the world.

In the United States, you'll generally find three types of summer squash:

Zucchini, whose skin can be yellow in color but is much more often found in grocery stores showcasing its dark green skin. (The dark green skin of zucchini may also be naturally striped or speckled.) Zucchini is one of the summer squash types that grow on flowering plants with edible flowers.

Black beauty, cocozelle, golden, courgette, and dark green are some of the popular varieties of zucchini.

Crookneck and straightneck squashes, usually yellow in color. While sometimes available with light green skins, bright yellow crookneck and straightneck squashes are the varieties that we most commonly associate with summer squash. (We've become especially accustomed to seeing small, bulb-shaped, bright yellow crookneck squashes in the United States.) Crookneck and straightneck summer squashes can be very similar in appearance, since crookneck varieties may have a very minimally curved neck that is almost swan-like in appearance. Golden summer, yellow crookneck, and early straightneck are some popular varieties of crookneck and straightneck squashes. Cushaw squashes are special varieties of crookneck squashes that are much larger than other crooknecks, even though they are easily recognized by their similar bulb-like shape. Cushaws take about twice as long to grow as other crooknecks, and are often used in baking (for example, in pies).

Scallop squashes, also called pattypan squashes. These summer squashes are typically saucer-shaped and come in a wide variety of colors from very pale yellow to golden yellow to medium green. Scallop squashes sometimes have a slightly sweeter flesh than other summer squashes. Popular varieties include green tint scallop, scallop early white bush, scallop yellow bush, and sunburst. In some countries, you'll also hear the words "scallopini" or "button squash" used to describe the scallop squashes.

Health Benefits:

- Zucchini is one of the very low calorie vegetables. It contains no saturated fats or cholesterol. Its peel is good source of dietary fiber that helps reduce constipation and offers some protection against colon cancers.

- Zucchinis have anti-oxidant value (Oxygen radical absorbance capacity- ORAC) the value which is far below to some of the berries, and vegetables. Nonetheless, the pods are one of the common vegetables included in weight reduction and cholesterol control programs by the dieticians.

- Furthermore, zucchinis, especially golden skin varieties, are rich in flavonoid poly-phenolic antioxidants such as *carotenes, lutein and zea-xanthin.* These compounds help scavenge harmful oxygen-derived free radicals and reactive oxygen species (ROS) from the body that play a role in aging and various disease processes.

- Courgette is a relatively moderate source of folates. Folates are important in cell division and DNA synthesis. When taken adequately before pregnancy, it can help prevent neural tube defects in the fetus.

- It is a very good source of potassium, an important intra-cellular electrolyte. Potassium is a heart friendly electrolyte and helps bring the reduction in blood pressure and heart rates by countering pressure-effects of sodium.

- Fresh fruits are rich in vitamin A.
- Fresh pods, indeed, are good source of anti-oxidant vitamin-C.
- In addition, they contain moderate levels of B-complex group of vitamins like thiamin, pyridoxine, riboflavin and minerals like iron, manganese, phosphorus, and zinc.

Selection and storage:

Zucchinis are available all around the year, but they are at their best during late spring and summer seasons.

In the stores choose small to medium-sized zucchini featuring shiny, bright green skin, firm and heavy in hand. The best size for zucchini is 6 to 8 inches long and 2 inches or less in diameter. Some big sized varieties with marrow are specially grown especially for stuffing. Minor superficial scratches and mild bruises are oftentimes seen on their surface but are perfectly fine.

Avoid overly mature, large courgette with pitted skin or those with flabby or spongy texture. Furthermore, avoid those with soft and wrinkled ends as they indicate old stock and state of de-hydration. Go for organically grown products to get rich flavor and nutrient content.

At home, place them in plastic bag and store inside the vegetable compartment of the refrigerator set with adequate moisture. They can be stored for up to 2-3 days.

Preparation:

Wash them thoroughly in cold, running water just before cooking. Sometimes the fruits may require light scrub at places where prickles or dirt attached firmly. Trim the neck and bases. Peeling of skin is not advised.

Zucchini blossoms are also an edible delicacy. In general, blossoms are picked up during morning hours when they are fresh and soft. To prepare, open up blossoms and carefully inspect for insects. Pull off any calyces attached firmly at the base.

Some preparation ideas:

- Fresh, tender zucchini can be eaten raw in salads.
- The pods can be used fried, baked, steamed, boiled, or used in stuffing.
- It mixes well with potatoes, carrots, asparagus, green beans, etc., in stews, sabzi, and curries.
- Fine-sections, chopped or grated, it can be shredded into bread, pizza, etc.

SWISS CHARD
OR SILVER BEET AS GREENS

Chard is a tall leafy green vegetable commonly referred to as Swiss chard and scientifically known as *Beta vulgaris*. Chard belongs to the same family as beets and spinach and shares a similar taste profile with a flavor that is bitter, pungent, and slightly salty. Swiss chard is truly one of the vegetable valedictorians with its exceptionally impressive list of health-promoting nutrients. Although Swiss chard is available throughout the year, its peak season runs from June through August when it is at its best and in the greatest abundance at your local supermarket.

Swiss chard—along with kale, mustard greens and collard greens—is one of several leafy green vegetables often referred to as "greens". It is a tall leafy green vegetable with a thick, crunchy stalk that comes in white, red or yellow with wide fan-like green leaves.

Chard has a thick, crunchy stalk to which fan-like wide green leaves are attached. The leaves may either be smooth or curly, depending upon the variety, and feature lighter-colored ribs running throughout. The stalk, which can measure almost two feet in length, comes in a variety of colors including white, red, yellow and orange. Sometimes, in the market, different colored varieties will be bunched together and labeled "rainbow chard."

We've become accustomed to thinking about vegetables as great sources of phytonutrients. Indeed they are! But we don't always appreciate how unique each vegetable can be in terms of its phytonutrient content. Recent research has shown that chard leaves contain at least 13 different polyphenol antioxidants.

These are leaflets or mid-ribs of the white beet. Take them while young and tender, wash, tie into bundles, boil and dress precisely the same as asparagus on toast. Serve with them, sauce Hollandaise or English drawn butter.

This makes one of the most delicate and delicious of dishes.

Swiss chard comes in variety of types based on their shiny, crunchy stalks and petiole:

- Green stalk: *Lucullus.*
- Red stalk: *Charlotte, Rhubarb Chard.*
- Multi-color stalk: Bright lights (white, orange, yellow, purple, pink)

Health Benefits:

- Swiss chard, like spinach, is the store-house of many phytonutrients that have health promotional and disease prevention properties.
- Chard is very low in calories and fats, recommended in cholesterol controlling and weight reduction programs.
- Chard leaves are an excellent source of antioxidant vitamin, vitamin-C. As a powerful water-soluble antioxidant, vitamin C helps to quench free radicals and reactive oxygen species (ROS) through its reduction potential properties. Research studies suggest that regular consumption of foods rich in vitamin C help maintain normal connective tissue, prevent iron deficiency, and also help the human body develop resistance against infectious agents by boosting immunity.
- Chard is one of the excellent vegetable sources for vitamin-K. Vitamin K has potential role bone health by promoting osteotrophic (bone formation

and strengthening) activity. Adequate vitamin-K levels in the diet help limiting neuronal damage in the brain; thus, has established role in the treatment of patients suffering from Alzheimer's disease.

- It is also rich source of omega-3 fatty acids; vitamin-A, and flavonoids anti-oxidants like ß-carotene, α-carotene, lutein and zea-xanthin. Carotenes convert to vitamin A inside the body.

- It is also rich in B-complex group of vitamins such as folates, niacin, vitamin B-6 (pyridoxine), thiamin and pantothenic acid that are essential for optimum cellular metabolic functions.

- It is also rich source of minerals like copper, calcium, sodium, potassium, iron, manganese and phosphorus. Potassium is an important component of cell and body fluids that helps controlling heart rate and blood pressure by countering effects of sodium. Manganese is used by the body as a co-factor for the antioxidant enzyme, *superoxide dismutase*. Iron is required for cellular oxidation and red blood cell formation.

Regular inclusion of chard in the diet has been found to prevent *osteoporosis, iron-deficiency anemia, and vitamin-A deficiency*; and believed to protect from cardiovascular diseases and colon and prostate cancers.

Selection and storage:

Swiss chard is available at its best during summer months from June until October. Chard can be harvested while its leaves are young and tender or after maturity when the leaves are larger and attained slightly tougher stems. In the store, buy fresh chard leaves featuring crispy, crunchy, brilliant dark-green color.

Chard is an extremely perishable leafy vegetable, and for the same reason it should be used as early as possible once harvested. If at all to store inside the refrigerator, then, set its temperature below 35 degree F and high humidity level to retain vitality for 1-2 days.

Preparation:

As in spinach, chard leaves should be washed thoroughly in clean running water and rinsed in saline water for about 30 minutes in order to remove soil, dirt and any insecticide/fungicide residues.

Some preparation ideas:

- Fresh young chard leaves can be used raw in salads.
- Mature chard leaves and stalks are typically cooked, braised or sautéed; the bitter flavor fades with cooking. However, antioxidant properties of chard are significantly decreased on steaming, frying and boiling.

Safety Precaution:

- Because of its high vitamin K content, patients on anti-coagulant therapy such as warfarin are encouraged to avoid this food since it increases the vitamin K concentration in the blood, which is what the drugs are often attempting to lower. This effectively raises the dose of the drug and causes toxicity.
- Swiss chard contains oxalic acid, a naturally-occurring substance found in some vegetables, which may crystallize as oxalate stones in the urinary tract in some people. It is, therefore, advisable to avoid eating chard in people with known oxalate urinary tract stones. Adequate intake of water is therefore advised to maintain normal urine output.

TOMATOES
(*Lycopersicum esculentum*, Miller)

The French sometimes refer to the tomato as pomme d'amour, meaning "love apple," and in Italy, tomato is sometimes referred to as "pomodoro" or "golden apple," probably referring to tomato varieties that were yellow/orange/tangerine in color.

Regardless of its name, the tomato is a wonderfully popular and versatile food that comes in over a thousand different varieties that vary in shape, size, and color. There are small cherry tomatoes, bright yellow tomatoes, Italian pear-shaped tomatoes, and the green tomato, famous for its fried preparation in Southern American cuisine.

Well ripened tomatoes contain nearly ninety per cent, of water; in the remaining ten per cent, there is a very little pectose and mineral matter, not enough, however, to give a food value. Authorities disagree as to whether or not tomatoes are wholesome. Of one thing we are quite sure, they are detrimental to persons who have oxahiria or uric acid diathesis.

Tomatoes are a treasure of riches when it comes to their antioxidant benefits. In terms of conventional antioxidants, tomatoes provide an excellent amount of vitamin C and beta-carotene; a very good amount of the mineral manganese; a good amount of vitamin E; and phytonutrients.

Tomatoes are capable of great variation in cooking, hence, are exceedingly popular. There is no doubt, however, that they are more easily digested raw, seasoned with a little olive oil, salt and pepper, or salt and pepper alone. Containing oxalic combined with malic acid, they are sufficiently acid without the addition of vinegar. Served persistently with salt, pepper and vinegar they will produce ulcerations of the mouth and intestinal disturbances. Unripe they are used for stuffing, pickling and preserving.

Health Benefits:

- Tomatoes are one of the low-calorie vegetables. They are also very low in any fat contents and have zero cholesterol levels. Nonetheless, they are excellent sources of antioxidants, dietary fiber, minerals, and vitamins. Because of their all-round qualities, dieticians and nutritionists often recommend them to be included in cholesterol controlling and weight reduction programs.

- The antioxidants present in tomatoes are scientifically found to be protective of cancers, including colon, prostate, breast, endometrial, lung, and pancreatic tumors.

- Lycopene, a flavonoid antioxidant, is the unique phytochemical present in the tomatoes. Red varieties are especially concentrated in this antioxidant. Together with carotenoids, it can protect cells and other structures in the body from harmful oxygen-free radicals. Studies have shown that *lycopene* prevents skin damage from ultra-violet (UV) rays and offers protection from skin cancer.

- Zea-xanthin is another flavonoid compound present abundantly in this vegetable. Zea-xanthin helps protect eyes from "age-related macular related macular disease" (ARMD) in the elderly persons by filtering harmful ultra-violet rays.

- The vegetable contains very good levels of vitamin A, and flavonoid anti-oxidants such as α and ß-carotenes, xanthins and lutein. Altogether, these pigment compounds are found to have antioxidant properties and take part in vision, maintain healthy mucus membranes and skin, and bone health. Consumption of natural vegetables and fruits rich in flavonoids is known to help protect from lung and oral cavity cancers.

- Additionally, they are also good source of antioxidant vitamin-C; consumption of foods rich in vitamin C helps the body develop resistance against infectious agents and scavenge harmful free radicals.
- Fresh tomato is very rich in potassium. Potassium is an important component of cell and body fluids that helps controlling heart rate and blood pressure caused by sodium.
- Further, they contain moderate levels of vital B-complex vitamins such as folates, thiamin, niacin, riboflavin as well some essential minerals like iron, calcium, manganese and other trace elements.

Selection and storage:

Fresh ripe fruits feature beautiful bright-red color and have a rich fruity flavor. In the markets, buy fresh, firm, uniform sized fruits. Avoid those with wrinkle surface, discolored spots, cuts and too soft and mushy.

Firm, yellow fruits can be placed in cool, dark place at room temperature for 2-3 days. However, ripe tomatoes are one of the easily perishable vegetables and should be stored in the refrigerator. Use them while they are fresh to obtain full benefits of vitamins and antioxidants.

Preparation:

Pests are common in tomatoes. Hybrid varieties are usually subjected to insecticide spray. Therefore, wash them thoroughly in the cold running water in order to remove dust, soil and any insecticide/fungicide residues.

To prepare, discard stem and top calyx end and cut into desired halves, cubes, slices, etc. Peel the skin and puree its juicy pulp. Some prefer to de-seed the fruit before adding in cooking.

Some preparation ideas:

- They are used extensively in cooking especially in Mediterranean, Greek, Italian, Southeast Asian, and East European cuisine.
- Raw ones have extra acidic taste, but when mixed with other ingredients while cooking gives wonderful flavor and rich taste.
- Regular as well as cherry tomatoes are one of the popular items in salad preparations.
- Fresh tomato juices as well as its soups are increasingly becoming popular health-drinks all across the world. Organic varieties contain three times the more lycopene than non-organic.
- Unripe green tomatoes are used in many similar ways like other raw vegetables to prepare in curries, stews and to make "chutney" in some of the Indian subcontinent states.

Safety Precaution:

Allergic reactions to tomatoes may sometimes occur with symptoms like skin and itching eyes, runny nose, gastrointestinal disturbances like pain abdomen, vomiting and diarrhea.

TURNIPS

The most common type of turnip is mostly white-skinned apart from the upper 1–6 centimeters, which protrude above the ground and are purple, red, or greenish wherever sunlight has fallen. This above-ground part develops from stem tissue, but is fused with the root. The interior flesh is entirely white. The entire root is roughly conical, but can be occasionally global, about 5–20 centimeters in diameter, and lacks side roots. The taproot (the normal root below the swollen storage root) is thin and 10 centimeters or more in length; it is trimmed off before marketing. The leaves grow directly from the above-ground shoulder of the root, with little or no visible crown or neck (as found in rutabagas).

Of these we have two varieties, *Brassica campestris*, Linn., the ruta-baga or Swedish turnip, and *Brassica Rapa*, Linn., the white turnip. The Swedish turnip or ruta-baga is not so sweet, but slightly more nutritious than the common white turnip; both are prepared after the same recipes.

In chemical composition the turnip is very much like the cabbage, save that it contains a little more water and less nitrogenous matter. They do not contain either sugar or starch. The carbohydrates are presented in the form of *inulin* and *pectose*, which make them an agreeable and harmless vegetable for diabetic persons, provided they are cooked carefully and served with salt, pepper and butter only.

Turnip tops or sprouts of the old turnips, are boiled as greens, or served raw as a spring salad. When well prepared, they are quite palatable.

Health Benefits:
- Turnips are very low calorie root vegetables. However, they are very good source of anti-oxidants, minerals, vitamins and dietary fiber.
- Fresh roots are indeed one of the vegetables rich in vitamin C. Vitamin-C is a powerful water-soluble anti-oxidant required by the body for synthesis of collagen. It also helps the body scavenge harmful free radicals, prevents from cancers, inflammation, and helps boost immunity.
- Turnip greens indeed are the storehouse of many vital nutrients; contain certain minerals and vitamins several fold more than that in the roots. The greens are very rich in antioxidants like vitamin A, vitamin C, carotenoid, xanthin, and lutein. In addition, the leafy-tops are an excellent source of vitamin K.
- In addition, its top greens are also a very good source of B-complex group of vitamins such as folates, riboflavin, pyridoxine, pantothenic acid and thiamin.

- Furher, the fresh greens are also excellent sources of important minerals like calcium, copper, iron and manganese.

Selection and storage:

Turnips are available year around; however, fresh roots are abundant in October through March. At maturity, they are usually two to three inches in diameter and weigh between 60 to 250 g.

This root vegetable usually sold bunched or topped. In the markets look for fresh roots that are small, firm, round and impart delicate sweet flavor. Avoid larger as well as over matured roots as they are woody in textured and excess in fiber that makes dishes unappetizing.

Once at home, remove the top greens as they rob nutrients of the roots. The roots can be stored for few weeks at low temperatures (32°-35° F) and high relative humidity (95 percent or above). Use top greens as early as possible as they lose nutrients rather quickly.

Preparation:

Both root and top greens are used for cooking. Wash roots in cold running water in order to remove soil and any fungicide residues from the surface. Trim the top and bottom ends of the vegetable. Peeling may not be necessary if roots are young; however, over matured turnips will have tough skin that should be removed.

Some preparation ideas:

- Young turnips are one of the favored items in raw salads for their sweet taste, complementing with cabbage, parsnips, carrots, beets, etc.
- Its cubes can mix well with other vegetables like kohlrabi, potato, carrots in variety of stews.
- Diced roots can be added to poultry, lamb, pork, etc.
- Add raw baby turnip slices with olives and cherry tomatoes to make delicious appetizer.
- Turnip cubes are pickled as in other vegetables like radish, chili-peppers, carrot in many parts of Northern India, Iran, and Pakistan.
- Top greens are used with other greens and vegetables in soups, curries, and stews.

Safety Precaution:

Turnips and top greens are generally very safe, including in pregnant women.

However, the roots and top greens contain small amount oxalic acid, a naturally-occurring substance found in some vegetables belonging to Brassica family, which may crystallize as oxalate stones in the urinary tract in some people. It is therefore, those with known oxalate urinary tract stones may have to avoid eating them. Adequate intake of water is advised to maintain normal urine output in these individuals to minimize the stone risk.

VEGETABLE MARROW
(*Cucurbifa Ovifera*, Linn.)

Marrow vegetable is a general term used to refer to a number of summer squash varieties. Also known in the United Kingdom as vegetable marrows or simply marrows, marrow vegetables are typically larger and longer than zucchini, with smooth, thin, edible peel that can range in color from light beige to deep green. Marrow vegetables have a mild flavor that lends easily to both simple and complex dishes.

They are extensively cultivated in England, but little known in the United States.

Cook and serve according to the rules for cucumbers.

A GROUP OF SALAD PLANTS

Arugula
Chicory
Corn Salad or Lamb's lettuce
Endive
Garden Cress or Pepper Grass
Lettuce
Mustard
Radicchio
Water Cress

Although some of the plants in this group are frequently cooked, they are decidedly more palatable and attractive when served raw. They are quite free from sugar and starch; are very succulent, containing from 90 to 95 per cent, water, and a small amount of mineral matter. A few contain pungent volatile oils to which they owe their flavor.

ARUGULA

Arugula is a nutritious green-leafy vegetable of Mediterranean origin. It belongs within the *Brassicaceae* family similar as mustard greens, cauliflower, kale...,etc.

Arugula is a small, low growing annual herb featuring dandelion like succulent, elongated, lobular leaves with green-veins. In young plant, however, the plain light green leaves appear identical to that of spinach. Young, tender leaves feature sweet, nutty, flavor and less peppery taste in contrast to strong, spicy flavor of mature greens.

Health Benefits:

- As in other greens, arugula is one of very low calorie vegetable. 100 g of fresh leaves provides just 25 calories. Nonetheless, it has many vital phytochemicals, anti-oxidants, vitamins, and minerals that can immensely benefit health.

- Arugula salad is a rich source of certain phytochemicals such as *indoles, thiocyanates, sulforaphane*, and *isothiocyanates*. Together, they have been found to counter carcinogenic effects of estrogen and thus help benefit against prostate, breast, cervical, colon, ovarian cancers by virtue of their cancer-cell growth inhibition, cytotoxic effects on cancer cells.

- In addition, *di-indolyl-methane (DIM),* a lipid soluble metabolite of indole has immune modulator, anti-bacterial and anti-viral properties. DIM has currently been found as an application in the treatment of recurring respiratory papillomatosis,

- Arugula is a very good source of folates. When given to the anticipant mothers during their conception time, folate helps prevent neural tube defects in the newborns.

- Arugula is an excellent source of vitamin A. Studies found that vitamin A and flavonoid compounds in green leafy vegetables help protect from skin, lung and oral cavity cancers.

- This vegetable also rich in B-complex group of vitamins such as thiamin, riboflavin, niacin, vitamin B-6 (pyridoxine), and pantothenic acid those are essential for optimum cellular enzymatic and metabolic functions.
- Fresh arugula leaves contain good levels of vitamin C. Vitamin C is a powerful, natural anti-oxidant.
- Arugula is one of the excellent vegetable sources for vitamin-K. Vitamin K has potential role bone health by promoting osteotrophic (bone formation and strengthening) activity. Adequate vitamin-K levels in the diet help limiting neuronal damage in the brain; thus, has established role in the treatment of patients suffering from *Alzheimer's disease*.
- Arugula leaves contain adequate levels of minerals, especially copper and iron. In addition, it has small amounts of some other essential minerals and electrolytes such as calcium, iron, potassium, manganese, and phosphorus.

Selection and storage:

Fresh arugula is available in the markets all year. When buying, look for crispy green color young leaves. Avoid flowered harvest, as its leaves are tough and bitter in taste. Discard any bruised, slump leaves and stems before storage.

Store the herb as you do for other greens like spinach, kale, etc. Place it in the vegetable compartment of the refrigerator set at high relative humidity.

Preparation:

Field grown arugula may is often sold in the local markets with root attached. Cut open the bushel and trim the lower stems. Discard yellow, wilted, bruised leaves. Place the leaves in a large bowl of cold water and swish thoroughly as you do it in cases of other greens like spinach in order to remove sand, soil, dirt...etc. Then drain the water, gently pat dry using moisture absorbent cloth before use in cooking.

Young tender arugula leaves can be added to salads and sandwiches. Fresh greens are used in soups, stews, juices and cooked as a vegetable.

CHICORY
(*Cichorium Intybus*, Linn.)

Chicory very nearly resembles the well bleached endive, except that the leaves are tiny, split and very sweet. It is one of the best of winter salad materials; it may be served alone, eaten with salt, in place of celery, or dressed with French dressing and served as a dinner salad.

The roots are sliced, dried, roasted, ground and used as an addition to coffee or as a coffee adulterant. Many cheap ground coffees are largely chicory. A little finely powdered chicory root mixed with a good coffee improves the infusion, but the mixing should be done at home; coffee is expensive and chicory cheap.

CORN SALAD OR LAMB'S LETTUCE
(*Valerianella olitoria*, Poll.)

This plant grows wild in Southern Europe, and is cultivated in the eastern part of the United States for early spring salads. It comes just between the winter and spring lettuce. The size and flavor of the leaves are greatly improved by cultivation.

ENDIVE
(*Cichorium Endizna*, Linn.)

The delicate white endive, with French dressing, makes one of the most delightful dinner salads and may also be wilted the same as dandelions.

This plant is grown in late summer and fall for a winter salad. When full grown the root leaves are tied up in a bunch, covered with boards and earth and bleached the same as celery. When well bleached, curly and crisp makes an excellent salad. If not well bleached or too old for bleaching, it is bitter and unpalatable. Cut in two-inch lengths, mix with lettuce or celery, and serve with French dressing as a dinner salad. The outside green leaves are frequently cut into small pieces, boiled in salt water and served as greens.

There is a variety:

- Curly-endive or frisee with curly narrow leaves
- Escarole or scarole with broad leaves.
- Belgian endive with smooth cream-colored leaves compressed into a compact long head.

Health Benefits:

- Endive is one of the very low calorie leafy vegetable. 100 g fresh leaves provide just 17 calories; however, contains a good amount of fiber.
- Endive is enriched with good amount Vitamin A and ß-carotene. Both compounds are known to have antioxidant properties. Carotenes convert to vitamin A in the body. Furthermore, vitamin A is required for maintaining healthy mucus membranes and skin. In addition, it is also essential vitamin for good eye-sight. Consumption of natural vegetables/greens rich in vitamin A helps to protect from lung and oral cavity cancers.
- It contains good amounts of many essential B-complex groups of vitamins such as **folic acid**, pantothenic acid (vitamin B5), pyridoxine (vitamin B6) and thiamin (vitamin B1), niacin (B3). These vitamins are essential in the sense that body requires them from external sources to replenish and required for fat, protein, and carbohydrate metabolism.
- Additionally, escarole is a good source of minerals like manganese, copper, iron, and potassium. Manganese is used as a co-factor for the antioxidant enzyme, *superoxide dismutase*.

Potassium is an important intracellular electrolyte helps counter the hypertension effects of sodium.

Selection and storage:

Fresh endive is available year around in the markets. Choose crispy, tender leafy tops. Avoid tough, yellow discolored leaves.

Store greens in plastic bag inside refrigerator. It will stay fresh for 3-4 days.

Preparation:

Wash fresh endive in cool running water. Discard yellow or any discolored leaves. Remove tough lower ends. Chop the leaves using paring knife.

Blanching removes bitterness from the leaves and enhances their flavor. Blanching is generally done by avoiding sunlight. Cover the plants for 2-4 weeks with inverted bushel baskets or plastic plates.

Wash them thoroughly in cold water before use. Trim the stem end with a sharp knife.

Frisee is featured in the popular French salad Lyonnaise.

Escarole is used in salads, soups and in sautéed recipes.

Witloof is used raw in salads or braised and served in vegetable.

GARDEN CRESS OR PEPPER GRASS
(*Lepidimn sativum*)

This resembles, in flavor and appearance, the ordinary water cress. When old, the leaves become exceedingly pungent and are unfit to use alone. Sprinkled over cabbage or lettuce, they give just a little of the mustard flavoring without the irritating effect of the ground mustard. When young and tender, they may be used alone with French dressing for a dinner salad.

LETTUCE
(*Lacttica sativa*, Linn.)

The varieties of lettuce supply a wholesome, cooling, palatable and digestible dinner salad. It is occasionally cooked, although the flavor and palatability are spoiled. The head or cabbage lettuce and the cos or upright (Romaine) are the commonest forms sold in this country. The long leaves of the cos or Romaine are tied together, covered with boards and earth for the purpose of bleaching. The extra time spent in care of this variety makes it quite expensive compared to common head lettuce. Lettuce is the common green served with French dressing as a dinner salad. It is too light and delicate to be served with mayonnaise.

Here are some popular varieties grown around the globe:

1. *Butter-head*, with loose heads; it has a buttery texture. Butter head cultivars are most popular and widely grown in Europe.

2. *Chinese variety or celtuce*, generally have long, tapering, non-head forming, strong-flavored leaves unlike its Western counterparts. They are,

therefore, used preferred in stir fried dishes and stews.

3. *Crisp-head* variety forms tight, dense heads that resemble cabbage. They are generally the mildest form, valued more for their crunchy texture than flavor. Cultivars of the crisp head are the most familiar type used in the USA.

4. *Loose-leaf* variety features tender, delicate and fully flavored leaves with a loose bunch. This group includes green oak leaf, red oak leaf, valeria and lolla-rosa-types.

5. *Romaine-lettuce* grows in a long head of sturdy leaves with a firm rib almost reaching to the tip of the leaf. Cultivars of Romaine are also the most popular types in the USA.

6. *Summer Crisp* variety forms moderately dense heads with a crunchy texture; this type is intermediate between crisp-head and loose-leaf types.

Health Benefits:

- Lettuce leaves are one of the very low calorie green-vegetables. Nonetheless, they are the store house of many phyto-nutrients that have health promoting and disease prevention properties.

- Vitamins in lettuce are plentiful. Fresh leaves are an excellent source of several Vitamin A and beta carotenes. These compounds have antioxidant properties. Vitamin A is required for maintaining healthy mucus membranes and skin, and is also essential for vision. Consumption of natural fruits and vegetables rich in flavonoids helps to protect the body from lung and oral cavity cancers.

- It is a rich source of vitamin K. Vitamin K has a potential role in the bone metabolism where it thought to increase bone mass by promoting osteotrophic activity in the bone cells. It also has established role in Alzheimer's disease patients by limiting neuronal damage in the brain.

- Fresh leaves contain good amounts folates and vitamin C. Folates require for DNA synthesis and therefore, vital in prevention of the neural tube defects in-utero fetus during pregnancy. Vitamin C is a powerful natural antioxidant; regular consumption of foods rich in vitamin C helps the body develop resistance against infectious agents and scavenge harmful, pro-inflammatory free radicals.

- Zea-xanthin, an important dietary carotenoid in lettuce, is selectively absorbed into the retinal macula lutea, where it thought to provide antioxidant and filter UV rays falling on the retina. Diet rich in xanthin and carotenes is thought to offer some protection against *age-related macular disease (ARMD)* in the elderly.

- It also contains good amounts of minerals like iron, calcium, magnesium, and potassium, which are very essential for body metabolism. Potassium is an important component of cell and body fluids that helps controlling heart rate and blood pressure. Manganese is used by the body as a co-factor for the antioxidant enzyme, *superoxide dismutase*. Copper is required in the production of red blood cells. Iron is essential for red blood cell formation.

- It is rich in B-complex group of vitamins like thiamin, vitamin B-6 (pyridoxine), riboflavins.
- Regular inclusion of lettuce in salads is known to prevent osteoporosis, iron-deficiency anemia and believed to protect from cardiovascular diseases, ARMD, Alzheimer's disease and cancers.

Selection and storage:

In the store, choose leaves that feature crispy outlook, bright in color. Avoid sunken leaves with spots or discoloration.

Each variety of lettuce features a unique keeping quality; hence, different methods should be applied while storing. Romaine and loose leaf-lettuces should be washed, and any excess water removed before storing in the refrigerator. Butter-head need not be washed before storing.

Pack them in a plastic bag or store in the refrigerator. Romaine will stay fresh for up to seven days whereas, Butter-head and loose leaf-types for two to three days.

Preparation:

Remove any outer discolored leaves. Then trim off their bitterly tips. Chop the remaining leaf to a desired size and discard the bottom stem/root portion.

Wash leaves then in clean running water and soak in salt water for about half an hour in order to remove sand and any parasite eggs and worms. Pat dry or use a salad spinner to remove the excess water.

Regardless of the type, all lettuces should feature crispy, fresh leaves that are free of dark or slimy spots. Varieties such as romaine and butter-head should have compact heads with no brown stems.

Raw, fresh-lettuce is commonly used in salads, sandwiches and spring rolls.

Chinese-lettuce is usually stir fried or stewed and added to noodles as well as fried rice preparations.

The leafy green also combines well with garden peas, green-beans as well as seafood like shrimp, prawns, etc.

MUSTARD

The young leaves of the *Brassica alba* are sweet and bland, and form an attractive spring salad. They do not contain any of the pungent oils found in the seeds. They may be mixed with corn salad, chicory or early spring lettuce, dressed with French or Italian dressing, and served as a dinner salad.

The mustard plant is native to sub-Himalayan plains of Indian sub-continent commonly cultivated for its winter season leaves and oil seeds since ancient times. Several cultivars exist. Mustards are winter crops when the leaves are more flavorful from November until March.

In general, its young tender green leaves that is harvested when the plant reaches about 2 feet in height and used as a green leafy vegetable. Completely grown plant reaches about 4-5 feet in height and bears golden yellow colored flowers.

Fresh mustards feature dark green colored broad leaves with flat surface and may have either toothed, frilled or lacy edges depending up on the cultivar type. Its light-green stem branches out extensively into many laterals.

Health Benefits:
- Mustard greens, like spinach, are the storehouse of many phyto-nutrients that have health promotional and disease prevention properties.
- Mustards are very low in calories and fats. However, its dark-green leaves contain a very good amount of fiber that helps control cholesterol level by interfering with its absorption in the gut. Additionally, adequate fiber in the food aids in smooth bowel movements and thereby offers protection from hemorrhoids, constipation as well as colon cancer diseases.

- The greens are supposed to be one of the highest among leafy vegetables, which provide vitamin K. Vitamin K has found to have a potential role in bone mass building function by promoting osteo-trophic activity in the bone. It also has established role in Alzheimer's disease patients by limiting neuronal damage in the brain.

- Fresh leaves are also a very good source of folic acid. This water-soluble vitamin has an important role in DNA synthesis and when given before, and early pregnancy may help prevent neural tube defects in the newborn baby.

- Mustard greens are rich source of anti-oxidants flavonoids, indoles, sulforaphane, carotenes, lutein and zea-xanthin. Indoles, mainly *di-indolyl-methane (DIM)* and *sulforaphane* have proven benefits against prostate, breast, colon and ovarian cancers by virtue of their cancer-cell growth inhibition, cytotoxic effects on cancer cells.

- Fresh mustard leaves are an excellent source of vitamin-C. Vitamin-C (ascorbic acid) is a powerful natural anti-oxidant that offers protection against free radical injury and flu-like viral infections.

- Mustard leaves are also incredible sources of vitamin-A. Vitamin A is an essential nutrient for maintaining healthy mucus membranes and skin and is required for good eye-sight. Consumption of natural fruits rich in flavonoids helps to protect from lung and oral cavity cancers.

- Fresh mustard greens are an excellent source of several essential minerals such as calcium, iron, magnesium, potassium, zinc, selenium, and manganese.
- Regular consumption of mustard greens in the diet is known to prevent arthritis, osteoporosis, iron deficiency anemia and believed to protect from cardiovascular diseases, asthma and colon and prostate cancers.

Selection and storage:

Mustards are winter crops. In the markets, look for fresh mustard greens featuring crispy, dark-green leaves and should show vitality. Avoid sunken, spotted, or discolored leaves.

The leaves wilt soon if kept at room temperature; therefore, should be stored inside the refrigerator immediately. Although they can be stored for up to three days in the cold storage, fresh mustard greens should be used as soon as early as possible to get maximum nutrition.

Preparation:

Fresh leaves, flower buds, and stems are used in a variety of cuisines all over Asia and in Eastern Europe.

Before cooking, wash the leaves thoroughly in clean running water to remove sand and soil and then rinsed in saline water for about 30 minutes in order to remove surface dust, any insecticide residues. Trim away thick petioles and stems.

Fresh tender mustard greens are eaten raw either as salad or as juice.

In South Asian cuisines, mustard is generally stew fried or steam cooked and mixed with other green. Its pungent, peppery flavor is somewhat tamed by adding butter, tomato, garlic and onion to the recipes.

Safety Concern:

Like spinach, reheating of mustard green leftovers may cause conversion of nitrates to nitrites and nitrosamines by certain bacteria that thrive on prepared nitrate-rich foods. These poisonous compounds may be harmful to health.

Phytate and dietary fiber present in the mustard greens may interfere with the bioavailability of iron, calcium and magnesium.

Because of its high vitamin K content, patients taking anti-coagulants such as warfarin are encouraged to avoid this food since it increases the vitamin K concentration in the blood, which is what the drugs are often attempting to lower. This may advertently raise the effective-dose of the drug.

Mustards contain *oxalic acid*, a naturally-occurring substance found in some vegetables, which may crystallize as oxalate stones in the urinary tract in some people. It is therefore, people with known oxalate urinary tract stones are advised to avoid eating vegetables belong to Brassica family.

Mustard greens may also contain *goitrogens*, which may interfere with thyroid hormone production and can cause thyroxin hormone deficiency in individuals with thyroid dysfunction.

RADICCHIO

Radicchio is a quick growing Mediterranean red colored leafy vegetable. It is actually one of the varieties of leaf chicory used in salads in Veneto regions of Italy for centuries. Its wine-red succulent, bitter flavored leaves hold several unique compounds like lactucopicrin (intybin), zea-xanthin, vitamin K and several other vitamins, minerals and antioxidants.

Radicchio is a perennial, small cabbage like plant. It prefers cool weather supplanted with well draining, fertile, moisture rich soil. The crop is ready to harvest after about 75-90 days after seedling. Hot weather and inadequate watering might results in small, dense, and bolting heads. Well-grown radicchio features compact wine-red color leaves with prominent white veins about the size of a romaine leaves with prominent white veins about the size of romaine lettuce head.

Health Benefits:
- Radicchio, like other chicory class vegetables, is very low in calories.
- The bitter principle in the radicchio is lactucopicrin (intybin), a sesquiterpene lactone.

Lactucopicrin is a potent anti-malarial agent and has a sedative and analgesic (painkiller) effect.

- Its leaves are an excellent source of phenolic flavonoid antioxidants such as *zea-xanthin* and *lutein*. Zea-xanthin is a xanthophyll category of flavonoid carotenoid (yellow pigment) which concentrates mainly in the central retina in the eyes. Together with lutein, it helps protect eyes from *age-related macular disease* (ARMD) by filtering harmful ultra-violet rays.

- Fresh leaves contain moderate amounts of essential B-complex groups of vitamins such as folic acid, pantothenic acid (vitamin B5), pyridoxine (vitamin B6) and thiamin (vitamin B1), niacin (B3). These vitamins are essential in the sense that body requires them from external sources to replenish and required for fat, protein and carbohydrate metabolism.

- Fresh radicchio is one of the excellent sources of vitamin K. Vitamin K has a potential role in bone health by promoting osteotrophic (bone formation and strengthening) activity. Further, adequate vitamin-K levels in the diet help limiting neuronal damage in the brain; thus, has established role in the treatment of patients suffering from Alzheimer's disease.

- Further, it is an also good source of minerals like manganese, copper, iron, zinc, and potassium. Manganese is used as a co-factor for the antioxidant enzyme, *superoxide dismutase.* Potassium is an important intracellular electrolyte helps counter the hypertension effects of sodium.

Selection and storage:

At its natural habitat, radicchio is a cool-season vegetable. Although it is grown in some parts of USA, a majority of it is imported from the Mediterranean, especially from the Italy. Some of the varieties are grown and marketed around the year in California region.

If you grow in the home garden, ensure the edible head is blanched appropriately before harvest as in endives. In some parts, forced second growth (heads) are harvested, whereas the green, bitter, first heads discarded. To harvest, cut the round, compact head off the root and trim away all the outer copper-green leaves as in cabbage.

In the markets select fresh, compact, bright wine-red colored heads with prominent mid-ribs. Closely look for cracks, spots, or mechanical bruising on the leaves. Treviso and Chioggia should have tight, compact leaves, whereas Verona type features open, loose leaves.

At home, store inside the refrigerator set at temperature below 8 °C with relative humidity of around 90% for up to 2-3 weeks.

Preparation:

Radicchio is used mainly as leafy salad vegetable. Raw leaves have been sharp, pungent in flavor. Exposure to more intense daylight makes its leaves bitter, which is somewhat mellowed once cooked.

To prepare, trim the outer leaves as you do it in cabbage. Wash the head in cool running water. Cut the head into quarters, wedges, and use in cooking.

Radicchio is a favorite winter-season salad vegetable in Southern Europe. Raw leaves are eaten in Italy in salads. In the USA lightly stewed leaves are preferred.

Its chunks are grilled gently with olive oil, artichoke hearts and beans in a delicious salad.

Radicchio risotto and pasta are popular winter recipes in the Northern Italian region.

WATER CRESS
(*Nasturtium officinale*, R. Brown.)

This plant grows wild on constantly running streamlets, sometimes spreading over the entire surface of the water, stopping the flow of the stream. The entire young plant is eaten. It may be used as a garnish or served in salads. It is antiscorbutic, palatable and wholesome.

Water cress owes its flavor to a volatile oil which grows very pungent as the plant matures and blossoms. Mixed with young dandelion leaves or spring lettuce or with shredded cabbage, it is much better than when served alone.

Health Benefits:

- Peppery and tangy flavored cress is a storehouse of many natural phytonutrients like *isothiocyanates* that have health promotional and disease prevention properties.

- Cress is one of the very low-calorie green leafy vegetables and contains negligible amounts of fats. Being an antioxidant rich, fewer calories and low-fat vegetable it is often recommended in cholesterol controlling and weight reduction programs.

- Cress leaves and stem contains gluconasturtiin, a glucosinolate compound that gives the peppery flavor. Research studies suggest that the hydrolysis product of gluconasturtiin, 2-phenethyl isothiocyanate (PEITC), is believed to be cancer preventing by inhibition of phase I enzymes (*mono-oxygenases* and*cytochrome P450s*).

- Fresh cress has more concentration of ascorbic acid (vitamin C) than some of the fruits and vegetables. As an anti-oxidant, vitamin C helps to quench free radicals and reactive oxygen species (ROS) through its reduction potential properties. Lab studies suggest that regular consumption of foods rich in vitamin C help maintain normal connective tissue, prevent iron deficiency, and also help the body develop resistance against infectious agents by boosting immunity.

- It is one of the excellent vegetable sources for vitamin-K. Vitamin K has potential role bone health by promoting osteotrophic (bone formation and strengthening) activity. Adequate vitamin-K levels in the diet help limiting neuronal damage in the brain; thus, has established role in the treatment of patients suffering from Alzheimer's disease.
- Cress is also an excellent source of vitamin-A, and flavonoids anti-oxidants like ß carotene, lutein and zea-xanthin.
- It is also rich in B-complex group of vitamins such as riboflavin, niacin, vitamin B-6 (pyridoxine), thiamin and pantothenic acid that are essential for optimum cellular metabolic functions.
- Further, it is also rich source of minerals like copper, calcium, potassium, magnesium, manganese and phosphorus. Potassium is an important component of cell and body fluids that helps controlling heart rate and blood pressure by countering effects of sodium. Manganese is used by the body as a co-factor for the antioxidant enzyme, *superoxide dismutase*. Calcium is required as bone/teeth mineral and in the regulation of heart and skeletal muscle activity.

Regular inclusion of cress in the diet is found to prevent osteoporosis, anemia, and vitamin A deficiency and believed to protect from cardiovascular diseases and colon and prostate cancers.

Selection and storage:

Watercress is available year around. In the stores, purchase thick, broad, succulent and deep green colored fresh leaves. Fresh cress leaves should impart tangy peppery aroma when squeezed between thumb and index fingers.

In general, this green leafy herb best grows in aquatic environments; therefore, it should be washed in clean running water and then soaked in salt water for about half an hour in order to rid off parasite eggs and worms that thrive in aquatic conditions.

Fresh greens submerged in water and stored in the refrigerator where they keep well for up to 2-3 days.

Preparation:

Watercress gives a beautiful peppery flavor to recipes. Soak in cold water for few minutes to revive sunken leaves. Separate roots from leaves. Then, rinse once again in clean water and pat dry before using in cooking. Trim away thick fiber stems.

Some preparation ideas:
- Fresh cress sprigs used in green salads.
- The greens are used in many European cuisines in sandwiches and vegetable drinks.
- They are also used in the preparation of soups.
- Cress leaves can also be steamed and eaten as a vegetable.

Safety Precaution:

Buy watercress from known source of farms using clean running water. Cress from stagnant and polluted water may host to some harmful parasites like flukes and larvae.

Watercress contains 0.31 mg of oxalic acid per 100 g of leaves. Oxalic acid is a naturally-occurring substance found in some vegetables, which may crystallize as oxalate stones in the urinary tract in some people. It is therefore, people with known oxalate urinary tract stones are advised to avoid eating vegetables belong to Brassica family.

Being a Brassica family vegetable, cress may also contain goitrogens, which may interfere with thyroid hormone production and can cause thyroxin hormone deficiency in individuals with thyroid dysfunction.

A FEW EDIBLE WEEDS

Photos found at:
http://vegetables.healthyfoodseries.com/edible-weeds/

Sourdock
Sorrel
Poke shoots
Lambs' Quarters
Purslane
Shepherds' Purse
Dandelion
Wild Pepper Grass

Check out the site at:

SOURDOCK
(*Rumex crispus*, Linn.)

This common weed grows along the roadsides or in rich pasture fields in the northern, western and central western United States. It is called sour dock or long, curly-leafed dock to distinguish it from the shorter wide-leafed dock. It may be cooked and served according to the rules for spinach. It makes, however, a much more delicate green. As it grows in the early spring, it gives the ordinary farmer an accessible vegetable long before other garden greens are ready for use.

It is usually served with boiled salt beef or pork. This contains oxalic acid.

SORREL
(*Rumex Acetosella*, Linn.)

This is the common sheep sorrel, or sour grass, an exceedingly common weed in all parts of the United States. A similar variety, *Rumex Acetosa*, is cultivated as a spring vegetable. Both of these are used mixed with lettuce or chicory, dressed with French dressing as a dinner salad. It is also used for soups and sauces. Sorrel sauce is a common accompaniment to roasted or fricandeau of veal, or veal cutlets. All sorrel contains oxalic acid and oxalates in goodly quantity.

POKE SHOOTS

These are the young shoots of the *Phytolacca decandra*, also called scoke or pigeon berry weed. In Eastern Pennsylvania the young shoots form a common green in the early spring. They are sold in the markets in bundles, and are cooked and served the same as asparagus. They should never be taken over three inches long, and should show only a small tuft of leaves at the top. Older or larger than this they are poisonous. Wash thoroughly in cold water one hour, tie in bundles like asparagus, put into a kettle of boiling water, add a teaspoonful of salt and boil three-quarters of an hour. Put them on buttered toast after draining, heads all one way. Cover with drawn butter and serve.

LAMBS' QUARTERS
(*Chenopodium capitatum*, Watson)

This is one of the commonest of garden weeds, and is the most delicate of the so-called greens. It may be cooked after any of the recipes given for spinach.

Chenopodium album, or white goosefoot, is cultivated in England and by English gardeners in the United States, and is considered one of the finest of garden greens. These contain a very little oxalic acid.

PURSLANE
(*Portulacca oleracea*, Linn.)

Purslane is a hardy annual plant, a common weed in most gardens. It is much stronger and better when cultivated. Boiled in salted water it forms an admirable green. It may also be added to stews, and is used frequently for sauces to serve with boiled salted beef.

Pursley is widely grown in many Asian and European regions as a staple leafy vegetable. Its leaves appear thick, contain mucilaginous substance, and have a slightly sour and salty taste. Leaves and tender stems have a slightly sour, and salty taste. In addition to succulent stems and leaves, its yellow flower buds are also edible.

Purslane seeds, appear like black tea powder, are often used to make some herbal drinks.

Health Benefits:
- This wonderful green leafy vegetable is very low in calories and fats; nonetheless, it is rich in dietary fiber, vitamins, and minerals.
- Fresh leaves contain surprisingly more omega-3 fatty acids (α-linolenic acid) than any other leafy vegetable plant. Research studies show that consumption of foods rich in ω-3 fatty acids may reduce the risk of coronary heart disease, stroke, and help prevent the development of ADHD, autism, and other developmental differences in children.
- It is an excellent source of Vitamin A, one of the highest among green leafy vegetables. Vitamin A is a known powerful natural antioxidant and is essential for vision. This vitamin is also required to maintain healthy mucus membranes and skin. Consumption of natural vegetables and fruits rich in vitamin A is known to help to protect from lung and oral cavity cancers.
- Purslane is also a rich source of vitamin C, and some B-complex vitamins like riboflavin, niacin, pyridoxine and carotenoids, as well as dietary

minerals, such as iron, magnesium, calcium, potassium, and manganese.

- Furthermore, present in purslane are two types of betalain alkaloid pigments, the reddish *beta-cyanins* and the yellow *beta-xanthins*. Both pigment types are potent anti-oxidants and have been found to have anti-mutagenic properties in laboratory studies.

Selection and storage:

In the store, buy fresh and healthy-looking purslane; look carefully for mold, yellow or dark spots as they indicate inferior quality. Go for organic product whenever feasible.

Wash fresh leaves and stem in clean cold running water in order to remove any soil and insecticide/fungicide residues. After removing from water, mop it with soft cloth to remove any moisture in them before storing in the refrigerator.

Purslane can be kept in the refrigerator for about 3-4 days but should be eaten while the leaves are fresh and not wilted.

Preparation:

The stems and flower buds are also edible. Trim the tough stems near roots using a sharp knife. Cook under low temperature for a shorter period in order to preserve the majority of nutrients. Although antioxidant properties are significantly decreased on frying and boiling, its minerals, carotenes and flavonoids may remain intact with steam cooking.

Fresh, raw leaves can be used as salad and as vegetable juice.

Fresh, tender leaves are used in salads. Sautéed and gently stewed stems and leaves served as a side dish with fish and poultry.

It has also been used in soup and curry preparations and eaten with rice and ragi cake in many South Indian recipes.

Stew fried and mixed with other greens such as spinach and vegetables are favorite dishes among Asians.

Safety Precaution:

Purslane contains oxalic acid, a naturally-occurring substance found in some vegetables, which may crystallize as oxalate stones in the urinary tract in some people. It is therefore, people with known oxalate urinary tract stones are advised to avoid eating purslane and certain vegetables belonging to amaranthaceae and Brassica family. Adequate intake of water is therefore advised to maintain normal urine output.

SHEPHERDS' PURSE
(Capsella Bursa-Pastoris, Moench)

This is a common weed in waste places and takes its name from its little purse-shaped seed pod. It may be boiled and served the same as spinach.

DANDELION
(*Taraxacum officinale*, Weber)

It is scarcely worth while to describe this very common weed; almost every child is perfectly well acquainted with the early yellow flower of the dandelion. The young root leaves are gathered in the early spring and used raw as a salad; or they may be boiled and served as greens according to any of the recipes for spinach. The leaves grow bitter as they grow older. For this reason the young leaves only should be selected. Dandelions form one of the most wholesome of all greens. Containing, as they do, taraxacum, they are especially good for the liver. Dandelion roots are cut into slices, dried and used medicinally. In some parts of the West they are also toasted and used as a coffee substitute. Mixed with roasted wheat and barley, they form what is known as "poor man's coffee."

WILD PEPPER GRASS
(*Lepidium Virginicum*, Linn.)

This is a common weed growing by the road-sides, called by the country folk, wild mustard. The leaves are similar to those of the true mustard and make an excellent flavoring for salads. They contain just enough of the mustard flavor to be agreeable, without the irritating effects of ground mustard.

249

PLANTS USED AS SEASONINGS AND FLAVORINGS

Photos found at:
http://vegetables.healthyfoodseries.com/plants-for-sea...-and-flavoring/

Parsley
Chervil
Tarragon
Angelica
Capers
Nasturtium
Garlic
Shallot
Chives
Bay Leaves
Gumbo Filée Powder
Marjoram
Summer Savory
Sage
Sweet Basil
Thyme
Mint

Spices

Anise
Cardamom
Caraway
Coriander
Cumin Seed
Fennel
Dill
Cinnamon
Allspice
Cloves

Mustard Flour
Turmeric
Indian Curry Powder
Nutmeg
Mace
Pepper
Ginger
Flavoring
Vanilla

Check out the site at:

PARSLEY

Parsley (*Carum petroselinum*, Bentham) is one of the common plants used as a flavoring and garnish for both meats and vegetables. It should be served and eaten with the dish as it contains antiscorbutic qualities.

CHERVIL

Sweet chervil (*Myrrhis odorata*, Linn.), is a pungent, aromatic plant used as flavoring for salads and as a garnish to delicate meat dishes. It is easily cultivated.

TARRAGON
(*Artemisia Dracunculus*)

The green leaves of tarragon are mixed with lettuce and served with French dressing as a dinner salad.

They are also dried and used in powdered form and preserved in vinegar. Tarragon vinegar is commonly used for sour sauces or dressings.

ANGELICA
(*Archangelica officinalis*, Linn.)

The stem of this plant resembles rhubarb in size and texture. It is pressed and made into sweet wine and a cordial, called chart ruse. It is conserved as a sweetmeat, and used for the flavoring of puddings; it is also cut into tiny rings and mixed with candies.

CAPERS

These are the flower buds of *Capparis spinosa*, a trailing shrub grown largely in Southern Europe. The buds are packed in bottles and covered with vinegar. They are used as flavoring to sauces and salads.

NASTURTIUM
(*Tropceolum majus*, Linn.)

The fruit of the common garden nasturtium has a flavor similar to capers, and is frequently used as a substitute. It is also added to pickles as a preservative, and sometimes to spiced fruits. A half pint of nasturtiums added to a large jar of pickles will prevent mold. The flowers are used for sandwiches and as a garnish to summer salads.

GARLIC
(*Allium sativum*)

A very pungent member of the onion tribe. The small bulbs or "cloves" grow in large clusters. One *'clove" is sufficient to flavor a good-sized dish. Garlic vinegar is used in the place of common vinegar as a seasoning to salads.

SHALLOT OR ESCHALOT
(*Allium Ascalonicum*, Linn.)

Shallots are the minor members of the onion tribe. They are usually chopped or finely sliced and sprinkled over the top of salads. They are also used as a delicate flavoring for soups and sauces. They are sold in the eastern markets by the quart, and in appearance resemble the brown skinned onion "sets."
Health Benefits:

- Shallots have better nutrition profile than onions. On weight per weight basis, they have more anti-oxidants, minerals, and vitamins than onions.

- They are rich source of flavonoid anti-oxidants such as quercetin, kemferfol...etc. Further; they contain sulphur anti-oxidant compounds such as *diallyl disulfide, diallyl trisulfide* and *allyl propyl disulfide*. These compounds convert to allicin through enzymatic action following disruption of their cell surface while crushing, and chopping.

- Research studies show that *allicin* reduces cholesterol production by inhibiting the *HMG-CoA reductase* enzyme in the liver cells. Further, it also found to have anti-bacterial, anti-viral, and anti-fungal activities.

- Allicin also decreases blood vessel stiffness by releasing vasodilator chemical *nitric oxide* (NO) and thereby help bring a reduction in the total blood pressure. Further research studies suggest that allicin inhibit the platelet clot-formation in the blood vessels that helps decrease an overall risk of coronary artery disease (CAD), peripheral vascular diseases (PVD), and stroke.

- The phyto-chemical compounds *allium* and *Allyl disulfide* in onion have anti-mutagenic (protects from cancers) and anti-diabetic properties (helps lower blood sugar levels in diabetics).

- Shallots contain several fold more concentration of vitamins and minerals than in onions, especially vitamin A, pyridoxine, folates, thiamin, vitamin C etc. Pyridoxine (B-6) helps raises GABA chemical levels in the brain that help sooth nervous irritability. They also contain a good amount of Vitamin A. Vitamin A is a powerful antioxidant that helps protect from lung and oral cavity cancers.

- Further, they are also good in minerals and electrolytes than onions; particularly iron, calcium, copper, potassium, and phosphorus.

Selection and storage:

Fresh shallots are readily available during spring and early summer season. Wet and humid conditions hamper their flavor and storage life. In the supermarkets, however, they are available in fresh, frozen, canned, pickled, powdered, and dehydrated forms.

While buying, look for well-shaped, fresh, clean, well-formed bulbs with thin coppery-brown dry outer skin.

Like in onions, avoid those that show sprouting or signs of black mold (a type of fungal attack) as they indicate that the stock is old. In addition, poor-quality bulbs often have soft spots, moisture at their neck, and dark patches, which may all be indications of decaying.

Unlike onions, eschalots tend to perish early. At home, store them in cool dark place away from moisture and humid conditions where they keep fresh for several days. They can also keep well in the refrigerator; however, you should use them soon once you remove from the refrigerator since they tend to spoil if they kept at room temperature for a while.

Preparation:

Shallots have a mild pungent flavor. Unlike onions, their taste will not hit your sinuses, or burn the tongue. Unlike garlic, they have less of an impact on the breath.

To prepare: trim the ends using a paring knife. Then peel the outer 2-3 layers of skin until you find fresh thick pinkish-white whorls. They may be used as a whole, or you can slice or cut them into fine cubes/rings depending upon the recipe type in a way similar to onions. Being smaller, eschalots cook easily.

Fresh shallots are used in salads whole or chopped in cubes.

In much Asian cooking the bulbs are used liberally in the preparation of curries, gravy, chutney, soups, stews, and pastes.

Thinly sliced bulbs caramelized and served as a spicy garnish over burgers, grilled chicken, etc. in India and Pakistan.

Like in onions, they are one of the common ingredients in pasta, pizza, noodles, stew-fries, spice stuffing, etc.

Safety Precaution:

Although less in severity than onions, raw shallots can cause irritation to skin, mucus membranes, and eyes. This is due to release of *allyl sulfide* gas while chopping or slicing them which when comes in contact with wet surface becomes sulfuric acid. Allyl sulfide is concentrated more at the ends, especially at the root end. Its effect can be minimized by immersing the trimmed bulbs in cold water for a few minutes before you chop or slice them.

CHIVES
(*Allium Schanoprasum*, Linn.)

In appearance these resemble the wild or crow garlic, which grows in pastures in the early spring. They are sold in the markets, roots, bulbs and top, packed in small strawberry boxes. The green tops are washed, chopped and sprinkled over salads as flavoring.

BAY LEAVES
(*Laurus nobilis*, Linn.)

The dried leaves of this plant come to us from the district of the Mediterranean. The plant does not grow outside of the conservatories in America. The leaves can be purchased at any drug store; five or ten cents' worth will last a family of six for a year. They have a mild, peculiar aroma, and form a most acceptable flavoring for soups and stews.

GUMBO FILÉE POWDER

This is made from the very young leaves of the sassafras tree (*Sassafras officinale,* Nees) . Pick the first tiny leaves that come out in the spring, during the middle of a dry day. Spread them in the sun or in a moderately hot oven, to dry quickly. When perfectly dry rub them first in the hands, and then through a fine hair or wire sieve, and bottle for use. These leaves are very rich in mucilage, and are used as thickening to gumbo. Allow a teaspoon ful to each quart. The famous Brunswick stew of Virginia is also thickened with gumbo filée powder.

MARJORAM
(*Origanum majorana,* Linn.)

Marjoram (*Origanum majorana,* syn. *Majorana hortensis* Moench, *Majorana majorana* (L.) H. Karst) is a somewhat cold-sensitive perennial herb or undershrub with sweet pine and citrus flavors. In some Middle-Eastern countries, marjoram is synonymous with oregano, and there the names sweet marjoram and knotted marjoram are used to distinguish it from other plants of the genus *Origanum.*

SUMMER SAVORY
(*Satureia hortensis,* Linn.)

Summer savory (*Satureja hortensis*) is the better known of the savory species. It is an annual, but otherwise is similar in use and flavor to the perennial winter savory. It is used more often than winter savory, as winter savory is thought to have a slightly more bitter flavor.

SAGE
(Salvia officinalis, Linn.)

Sage is an herb from an evergreen shrub, Salvia officinalis, in the mint family. Its long, grayish-green leaves take on a velvety, cotton-like texture when rubbed (meaning ground lightly and passed through a coarse sieve).

Sage enhances pork, lamb, meats, and sausages. Chopped leaves flavor salads, pickles, and cheese. It is one of the most popular herbs in the United States.

SWEET BASIL
(Ocimum Basilicum)

Do not mistake this for the wild basil or mountain pink of this country. Sweet basil does not grow wild in the United States, but it is grown by gardeners as a kitchen or pot-herb.

All these herbs are used as seasonings to meat dishes and stuffings.

THYME

A delicate looking herb with a penetrating fragrance, thyme is an herb we should all take time to investigate and enjoy. And with about sixty different varieties including French (common) thyme, lemon thyme, orange thyme and silver thyme, this herb is sure to add some spice to your life.

Of this there are two varieties; the common thyme, *Thymus vulgaris*, or wild thyme, and the creeping thyme, *Thymus Serpyllum*, or garden thyme.

Thyme has a long history of use in natural medicine in connection with chest and respiratory problems including coughs, bronchitis, and chest congestion.

MINT
SPEARMINT
(*Mentha viridis*, Linn.)

This is also called meadow mint; it grows wild in most parts of the United States. It is used both fresh and dried. Chopped fine, mixed with vinegar and sugar, it forms the common mint sauce served with lamb. Bruised and boiled with syrup it is used for sherbets and punches. Conserved it is sold as a sweetmeat, the same as candied violets and rose leaves. It may be dried to use for sweets or preserved in vinegar for sauce and salads.

SPICES

ANISE
(*Pimpinella anisum*)

The seeds of this plant contain an essential oil used for the flavoring of cordials and punches.

CARDAMOM
(*Elettaria cardmnomum*)

The seeds of this plant are used as flavoring for pilau and many of the East Indian meat dishes. Ground, they are one of the ingredients of curry powder.

CARAWAY
(*Carum Carui*, Linn.)

Caraway is one of the oldest spices and is known for not only its culinary uses, but is also of equal importance in medicine, cosmetics and perfumery. It belongs to the plant family *Umbelliferae* or also called as *Apiaceae*. The *Umbelliferae* is one of the great families of flowering plants, and contains about 300 genera with three thousand species of perennial, biennial or annual herbs, generally native to the temperate zones

CORIANDER
(*Coriandrum sativum*, Linn.)

Coriander is considered both an herb and a spice since both its leaves and its seeds are used as a seasoning condiment. Fresh coriander leaves are more commonly known as cilantro and bear a strong resemblance to Italian flat leaf parsley. This is not surprising owing to the fact that they belong to the same plant family (*Umbelliferae*).

The fruit of the coriander plant contains two seeds which, when dried, are the parts that are used as the dried spice.

When ripe, the seeds are yellowish-brown in color with longitudinal ridges. They have a fragrant flavor that is reminiscent of both citrus peel and sage. Coriander seeds are available in whole or ground powder form.

Coriander seeds have a health-supporting reputation that is high on the list of the healing spices. In parts of Europe, coriander has traditionally been referred to as an "anti-diabetic" plant. In parts of India, it has traditionally been used for its anti-inflammatory properties. In the United States, coriander has recently been studied for its cholesterol-lowering effects.

CUMIN-SEED
(*Cuminuin cyminum*)

Although the small cumin seed looks rather unassuming, it packs a punch when it comes to flavor, which can be described as penetrating and peppery with slight citrus overtones. Cumin's unique flavor complexity has made it an integral spice in the cuisines of Mexico, India and the Middle East.

Cumin seeds resemble caraway seeds, being oblong in shape, longitudinally ridged, and yellow-brown in color. This is not surprising as both cumin and caraway, as well as parsley and dill, belong to the same plant family (*Umbelliferae*). The scientific name for cumin is *Cuminum cyminum*.

Cumin is available both in its whole seed form and ground into a powder.

It is probably not just for taste alone that cumin has made it into the stellar ranks of Indian, Middle Eastern and Mexican cooking. This ordinary looking seed is anything but ordinary when it comes to health benefits.

FENNEL
(*Faniculum officinale*, Allioni)

The seeds of all these plants are used by the Germans as flavoring for cakes and breads. They are also greatly prized by the Orientals. Ground, they are the principal ingredients of curry powder; cumin-seeds are the chosen flavor for Dutch cheese.

Fennel is a versatile vegetable that plays an important role in the food culture of many European nations, especially in France and Italy. Its esteemed reputation dates back to the earliest times and is reflected in its mythological traditions. Greek myths state that fennel was not only closely associated with Dionysus, the Greek god of food and wine, but that a fennel stalk carried the coal that passed down knowledge from the gods to men.

Health Benefits:
- Fennel bulb is a versatile vegetable, used since ancient times for its nutritional and medicinal properties. This winter season has some noteworthy essential oils, flavonoid anti-oxidants, minerals, and vitamins that have known health benefits.

- Bulb fennel is one of very low calorie vegetables. 100 g bulb provides just 31 calories. Further, it contains generous amounts of fiber, very little fat and zero cholesterol.
- Fresh bulbs give sweet anise-like flavor. Much of it is due to high concentration of aromatic essential oils like *anethole, estragole, and fenchone (fenchyl acetate)*. Anethole has been found to have anti-fungal and anti-bacterial properties.
- The bulbs have moderate amounts of minerals and vitamins that are essential for optimum health. Their juicy fronds indeed contain several vital vitamins such as pantothenic acid, pyridoxine (vitamin B-6), folic acid, niacin, riboflavin, and thiamin in small but healthy proportions. 100 g fresh bulbs provide 27 µg of folates. Folic acid is essential for DNA synthesis and cell division. Their adequate levels in the diet during pregnancy can help prevent neural tube defects in the newborn babies.
- In addition, fennel bulb contains an average amount of water-soluble vitamin, vitamin-C. Vitamin C helps the body develop resistance against infectious agents and scavenge harmful, pro-inflammatory free radicals. Further, it has small amounts of vitamin A.
- The bulbs have very good levels of heart-friendly electrolyte potassium. It is an important electrolyte inside the cell. Potassium helps reduce

blood pressure and rate of heartbeats by countering effects of sodium. Fennel also contains small amounts of minerals such as copper, iron, calcium, magnesium, manganese, zinc, and selenium.

Selection and storage:

Fresh bulb fennels are readily available in early autumn or spring. However, they can be found much of the year. In the United States, the bulbs are labeled as "anise" in the markets, because of their anise like flavor.

To harvest, gently pull the whole plant off the ground firmly holding at the bulb base. Trim the roots and cut off the top green leafy stems as they rob nutrients from the fennel fronds.

In the stores, choose fresh pearly white fennel bulbs that are compact, heavy in hand, and attractive anise like sweet flavor. Buy medium-sized bulbs each weighing about 5-10 ounces.

Very large and over-mature bulbs are stringy and have a less intense flavor. Avoid dried out, shriveled bulbs and those with yellow discoloration, spots, splits, and bruised.

At home, place them in a zip pouch plastic bag and store inside the vegetable compartment of the refrigerator as you do in for leeks. They stay fresh for up to five days, however, prolong storage would make them lose some flavor.

Preparation:

Fennel bulb is used as a vegetable to add flavors to various dishes, particularly in salads, stews, and soups. Its blanched bulb has a unique aroma and a light, sweet, subtle licorice taste. The bulbs are one of the favorite winter season vegetables in whole of France and Italy.

To prepare, trim off the base as you do in onions. Cut away top leafy stalks just above the bulb. Remove tough outer one to two layers, as they are stringy and unappetizing or use them to prepare vegetable stock. Then the clear white bulb may be cut into cubes, sticks, or slices to add in recipes.

Thinly sliced raw finochhio is eaten alone, served with dip, or added to vegetable salads.

It can be steamed, braised, or sautéd and added in a variety of dishes.

Fennel bulb can be added to flavor meat, fish, pork, and poultry recipes.

DILL
(*Peucedanum gravcolcns*)

This plant resembles fennel; in fact, fennel is always used when dill cannot be obtained. Holland pickles, or Dutch cucumbers, are large cucumbers preserved in brine richly flavored with dill, and sold under the name of dill pickles.

Dill is a unique plant in that both its leaves and seeds are used as a seasoning. Dill's green leaves are wispy and fernlike and have a soft, sweet taste. Dried dill seeds are light brown in color and oval in shape, featuring one flat side and one convex ridged side. The seeds are similar in taste to caraway, featuring a flavor that is aromatic, sweet and citrusy, but also slightly bitter.

Dill's unique health benefits come from two types of healing components: *monoterpenes*, including carvone, limonene, and anethofuran; and *flavonoids*, including kaempferol and vicenin.

CINNAMON

True cinnamon consists of the dried inner bark of the tropical tree, *Cinnamomum zeylanicum*. This bark is thin, brittle and of a light brown color. Cinnamon is the mildest of all spices, and for this reason is used with delicate fruits, and as flavoring for cakes, as cinnamon bun and Spanish bun. Much of the low priced cinnamon is the bark of the cassia tree, another species of the same genus. Cassia is coarse and woody, and lacks the delicate flavoring of the true cinnamon. A "stick" of cinnamon is one piece of the bark, usually six or eight inches in length.

Cinnamon bark is widely used as a spice. It is principally employed in cookery as a condiment and flavouring material. It is used in the preparation of chocolate, especially in Mexico, which is the main importer of cinnamon. It is also used in many dessert recipes, such as apple pie, doughnuts, and cinnamon buns as well as spicy candies, tea, hot cocoa, and liqueurs. True cinnamon, rather than cassia, is more suitable for use in sweet dishes. In the Middle East, it is often used in savoury dishes of chicken and lamb. In the United States, cinnamon and sugar are often used to flavour cereals, bread-based dishes, and fruits, especially apples; a cinnamon-sugar mixture is even sold separately for such purposes. Cinnamon can also be used in pickling. Cinnamon bark is one of the few spices that can be consumed directly. Cinnamon powder has long been an important spice in Persian cuisine, used in a variety of thick soups, drinks, and sweets.

ALLSPICE

Pimenta (allspice) consists of the berry of the *Eugenia pimenta*, a tropical evergreen tree. This is sold both whole and ground. On account of the richness of flavor and its similarity to all the other spices, it is called "allspice."

CLOVES

Cloves are the dry flower buds of the *Eugenia caryophyllafa*. In purchasing cloves select those rich in oil and dark in color. Cloves being much more pungent than other spices, must be used sparingly.

MUSTARD FLOUR

The ground mustard, or mustard flour, is composed of both white and black mustard seeds. Some of the cheaper varieties are largely adulterated with cracker and bread crumbs; in fact, they have but a trace of mustard. The white seeds are pungent, but contain no essential oil. The black seeds contain an acrid substance, which when moistened is changed by the action of an *enzyme* (*myosin*) into a pungent essential oil, very hot and irritating. For this reason mustard is not used as a seasoning to delicate foods. Added to mayonnaise or French dressing it completely upsets the digestibility of the salad, besides spoiling or overpowering the delicate flavoring. Under all circumstances use it most cautiously, and under no conditions add it to the food for invalids or delicate children.

he German mustards, especially those sold in this country, consist of Rhine wine thickened with cornstarch, flavored with spices, and made pungent with black mustard. This mustard is less irritating than the ordinary home-made mustard.

The bright yellow mustards are, as a rule, colored with turmeric.

TURMERIC
(*Curcuma Longa*)

The rhizome of this plant is dried, ground and used as coloring (yellow), and flavoring for pickles and curry. In fact, it is the chief ingredient in curry powders. "Turmeric paper" is used for the determination of alkalies.

INDIAN CURRY POWDER

¼ pound of coriander seed
¼ pound of turmeric
2 ounces of cumin seed
2 ounces of fennel seed
½ ounce of mustard
½ ounce of cinnamon
½ ounce of Jamaica ginger
½ ounce of allspice
1 ounce of cardamom seed
10 small bay leaves

Grind and mix all the ingredients, except the bay leaves, cover, nd stand them aside overnight. Next morning, rub them through a fine hair or wire sieve, put the powder into bottles, mixing with it the bay leaves; cork sufficiently tight to completely exclude the air.

NUTMEG

These are the seed kernels of the *Myristica fragrans*, a handsome tropical evergreen tree. They are exceedingly rich in an essential, pungent oil. The fruit, in appearance, resembles a peach. After removing the flesh part, we come first to the seed coat, mace, then to the seed, which, when removed, gives us the kernel known as nutmeg. In preparation for the market, those kernels are rolled in lime to prevent the attack of insects. The short, round or "female" nutmegs are best; the "male" nutmeg is long, rather dry, and contains but little essential oil.

MACE

Mace is the accessory seedcoat to the nutmeg, and like it has a fixed, as well as an essential oil. The latter is more pungent in mace than in nutmeg. It is sold in the market both whole and ground, and is used as an ordinary spice. In removing the mace from the nutmeg, it is usually broken into halves, one of these pieces being called a "blade" of mace.

PEPPER
BLACK

Black pepper is made from the unripe berries of *piper nigrum*. The berries are picked when red, dried and then ground, shells and all. The whole berries are called "pepper corns."

WHITE

This is made from the ripe seed kernels of the same berry. The dark outside husk is rejected. Both white and black pepper contain an essential oil, and flavoring known as *peperin*. Of the two, the white is much more pungent.

Coarsely ground white pepper is called "mignonette" pepper.

GINGER
(*Zingiber officinale*, Linn.)

This plant is a native of both the East and the West Indies, where it is used as seasoning for nearly all sweet and made dishes. Our common ginger is the fleshy rhizome, dried and ground. These rhizomes also come to us in the early fall in a green condition, and are used by the housewife as flavoring to insipid fruits, as citron, melon, and water melon rind. It is also preserved, or crystallized, and served as a sweetmeat. The very young tender rhizomes are scraped, boiled in a syrup until perfectly clear, and are sold in our markets under the name of candied ginger "stems." They are more expensive than the common candied ginger, are sweeter, less pungent and less woody. The best ginger is that which comes from the Island of Jamaica. The dark integument is thoroughly scraped off the stems, and they are then dried and ground. For this reason, Jamaica ginger is known as "white ginger." This is much more expensive at first cost, than the common ground ginger, but onehalf the measure only need be used. Too much ginger hinders digestion. A small quantity used as seasoning, or a bit taken at the close of a meal, aids digestion, in preventing unnatural fermentations from springing up and overpowering the natural, weaker ones. For this reason curry powder, fresh or ground ginger, are a constant ingredient of meat dishes in the very hot climates. They stimulate digestion. If spices and high seasoning are ever to be recommended it certainly is in hot weather, when the digestion is rather sluggish.

FLAVORINGS

True flavorings are made from the essential oils of the fruits, seeds, or flowers, of the plants from which they take their names. Those bearing the name of the fruits, not containing essential oils, are called artificial flavorings. These are made from compound ethers, and colored to match their respective fruits. Bartlet pear, for instance, is a good example of an artificial flavoring. It is delightful, fragrant, but perfectly innocent of the fruit of which it bears the name. "Pineapple" flavor is another of this type, made from aldehyde, ethyl-butyrate, amylbutyrate, chloroform and glycerin. True vanilla is very accurately copied in the same way. These flavors are largely used for fruit jellies, jams, soda water and candies. Unfortunately, we do not know whether or not they are injurious; let them alone to make sure. Many flavorings can be made at home; in fact, the list is sufficiently large to remove the necessity of buying any form of extracts.

VANILLA

Vanilla is the fruit of *Vanilla planifolia*, a climbing orchid of Mexico and Central America. The fruit is in the form of a slender pod, from six to eight inches long, and dark in color. It owes its aroma to a substance called *vanillin*, which is now artificially made from some of the compound ethers, and also from *coniferin*, a substance found in the sapwood of the pines. On account of the accessibility and cheapness of the ethers, they are almost exclusively used in the preparation of cheap vanilla extracts.

Tonka bean, on account of the similarity of flavor, is a common adulterant. While it is mild and has an agreeable odor, to the *connoisseur* it is very unlike true vanilla. The aromatic flavor of a good vanilla bean is not lost in the cooking, while that of the cheap, artificial vanilla is easily dissipated. There is an aroma, but not that of true vanilla.

The delicate, much sought after flavor of the Philadelphia vanilla ice cream, is due to the cooking of the bean in a portion of the cream; or it may be rubbed with the sugar.

ORANGE FLAVORING

The flavoring of both orange and lemon is due to a volatile oil found in the yellow rind. Secure fully ripe, yellow oranges, grate off the thin yellow rind, and to each ounce allow a half pint of good alcohol. Put the two together in a fruit jar; shake them every day for a month; then filter and bottle for use.

Lemon Extract is made in precisely the same way.

BITTER ALMOND

Bitter almond is a variety of the common almond, the extract of which is used as flavoring for candies and white cakes. It should be used with great care, on account of the quantity of hydrocyanic acid it contains.

Peach leaves are frequently used by the country folk as flavoring for cakes. Put a few peach leaves on the cake cloth or rack, turn the cake out on the leaves, and allow it to remain until cold. It will have the most delicate flavor of bitter almonds.

ABOUT THE AUTHOR AND MORE FOR YOU

Rod Stone is the principle partner of **Rod Stone Group** and they focus on providing information on health, nutrition, and many other subjects to improve your life.

I began writing articles on health and nutrition in the mid '90s. In 2004 I started full time working with people and providing information and products to assist with health and nutrition. In 2008 I started to become involved with the importance of specialized high intensity workouts. In 2011 we became involved in Universal Energy and related fields.

Our nutritional and product site @ http://herbal-nutrition.net/rodstone has products and information on Weight Management, Fitness and Energy, Immune Solutions, Stress Management, Digestive Health, Women's Health, Men's Health, Children's Health, Healthy Aging and Sports Nutrition.

We have written dozens of books and hundreds of articles. We also have hundreds of websites to help people improve their life. You can find the links to these at: http://rodstonegroup.com/.

WE HAVE A SPECIAL FOR YOU!!!

At our media store we have over a thousand different books, audio and video products for your benefit. **We have a special for those that buy this book. Go to our media store at http://www.rodsmediastore.com/ and** *when you sign in you can send us a message with subject "Amazon" and our support staff will send you a reply and from then on all of your purchases will be at 50% off our sale prices.*

We also have great products to improve your life including many free ones at http://rsmediagrp.com/free-books/

We believe that "information is today's currency."

To your success,

Rod Stone Group

Rod has the following books and more currently listed in Amazon:

Mrs. Rorer's Vegetarian Cooking: Recipes from the Past & Scientific Proof from Today ~ Mrs. Rorer is considered to be America's first dietician based on her work in preparing healthy meals for the sick. She became a household name, which was uncommon for a woman during the period in which she lived.

Grow Your Vegetables for Your Nutritional and Financial Health ~ The food we eat, the clothes we wear, and the house which shelters us, are three great necessities of life. Of these three necessities, food is by far the most important. This is why we all need to grow as much of the vegetables that we eat as possible

Positive Thinking Learning the Important Art of Positive Thinking ~ If you are looking for understanding the Law of

Attraction, using advanced affirmations, the power of attraction and eliminating worry then this book on is for you.

Health Tips: Over 500 Tips for Your Health (part of the Healthy Food Series) ~ Every day we search for ways to feel better; this makes our days more enjoyable for ourselves as well as those around us. Health Tips provides you with a wide variety of quick, useful information.

www.ingramcontent.com/pod-product-compliance
Lightning Source LLC
Chambersburg PA
CBHW070849290526
45795CB00001B/49